the happy hormone tracker

*A Wellness Journal for Monthly Cycle Tracking
and Hormone Balance for Women*

· · ·

SHANNON LEPARSKI

welcome to the happy hormone tracker!

If you're here, it means you want to get to know your cycle in a more intimate way and are curious about tracking hormonal patterns. Well, you've come to the right place.

When you understand the patterns of your cycle, you can work with your flow, not against it.

This journal provides a safe space for you to track your hormonal rhythms—which goes far beyond just logging your period (although of course that's a big part of it!). As women, we have cyclical energies, moods, and abilities that fluctuate throughout the month and are connected to the cycles of nature. The phases of your cycle affect so much: how you feel, what you crave, the nutrients you need, how productive or motivated you are, the type of exercise you do, your mood, your fertility, and more. Getting in sync with these fluctuations is a transformative act of self-care.

〰〰〰〰〰

heads up

If you're on hormonal birth control—like the pill or an IUD with hormones—then parts of this tracker will not apply to you. This is because your birth control prevents you from going through natural hormonal fluctuations each month. Feel free to use it for tracking changes, habits, and moods, but you won't be able to track ovulation or a "real" menstrual bleed. If you're curious to learn more about how hormonal birth control affects you or how to go off of birth control, check out my book, The Happy Hormone Guide.

the four phases:

Let's start with the basics: the four phases of your cycle. Just like the lunar moon cycle, your body transitions through four phases about every 28-30 days, on average. Each phase invites a unique set of hormonal, physical, emotional, and psychological gifts. These are brief overviews to help you as you start tracking. If you're curious to learn more, my book *The Happy Hormone Guide* goes in-depth into each phase, including recommendations for improving symptoms and how to optimize each phase with recipes, beauty DIYs, supplements, supportive herbs, and more.

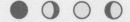

MENSTRUAL PHASE
winter/new moon: lasts 3-7 days

~~~~~~~~

The menstrual phase is the bleeding phase and is considered the winter season in your body. Consider it a chance to rest, conserve energy, and hibernate. This phase is believed to be a time when there is little distinction between intuition and logic, allowing you to gain deeper access to your inner wisdom and gut feelings. The bleeding phase is naturally cleansing (physically and emotionally), so while you may feel raw and sensitive, you are also letting go of what no longer serves you.

If you do not become pregnant, then 12 to 14 days after ovulation is when the corpus luteum (what's left of the egg follicle after the egg is released) stops making progesterone and gets reabsorbed in your body. This drop in progesterone is what triggers your uterus to contract and start your bleed. Day one of your period begins on the first day of heavy bleeding—not just light spotting. Tracking your first heavy day will help determine the length of your cycle, which lasts 3-7 days and gradually tapers off.

During this phase, hormones are at very low levels, which means you may have lower energy, your skin may look somewhat dry and dull, and you may feel more run-down than usual. This is generally the time to take it easy.

FOLLICULAR PHASE
spring/waxing moon: lasts 7-10 days

The follicular phase is the spring season in your body. It begins after your period ends and brings a sense of growth, renewal, and productivity—and an urge to plan. You may be able to see a clear path ahead and notice that life feels fresh and promising (which can be a nice change of pace after menstruation!).

This is the time when your body prepares to release an egg. Each ovary has hundreds of thousands of follicles (sacs of cells containing an immature egg at the center). In this phase, the pituitary gland is signaled to release FSH (follicle-stimulating hormone) to stimulate a number of follicles to grow (but only one will win and ovulate!). The maturing follicles release the hormone estradiol to thicken the uterine lining for implantation should the egg become fertilized.

This phase is all about increased energy, an awakened libido, elevated mood, and peak creativity. Because your brain chemistry is optimized at this phase, it's a great time to plan out your personal and work life. Think of it as your spring—a wonderful time for new beginnings and trying new things.

OVULATORY PHASE
summer/full moon: lasts 3-4 days

∿∿∿∿∿∿

The ovulatory phase is summer in your body. Life flows somewhat effortlessly in this phase. You may feel playful, flirty, and more outgoing than normal, which is ideal because this is when you're likely feeling your most beautiful! It's all about having fun, connecting with others, and allowing yourself to enjoy getting some extra attention.

Ovulation is the main event of your cycle overall. Typically, you are only fertile for 24 hours in your cycle (when the egg is released), but sperm can live inside you for up to five days (I know, right?) because they are nourished by your fertile cervical mucus, which has a stretchy, egg-white consistency. This is why tracking cervical mucus and basal body temperature is super important if you are trying to avoid pregnancy naturally (or get pregnant). Understanding when you are ovulating allows you to avoid intercourse, use protection, or time intercourse—depending on the outcome you're after.

Around day 12 of your cycle, the dominant follicle secretes a big surge of estrogen, prompting a flood of luteinizing hormone (LH). This causes the . . .

continued ⟶

O V U L A T O R Y   P H A S E *(continued)*

summer/full moon: *lasts 3–4 days*

~~~~~~~~~

...dominant follicle to grow rapidly until around day 14 (but varies for each woman), when the follicle finally ruptures and releases the egg. This is why you may feel a sharp twinge or cramping on one or both sides of your abdomen when you ovulate. (Another important thing to track.) Ovulation is a vital part of the menstrual cycle and is the only way your body is able to make progesterone in the next phase (the luteal phase).

During this phase, your skin may look extra glowy, the whites of your eyes may appear brighter, and you'll probably notice that you have lots of motivation and a high libido. (It's also when you are most fertile, so be careful!) You're also inclined to experience soaring energy to crush your workouts, too.

LUTEAL PHASE
autumn/waning moon: lasts 12–14 days

The luteal phase is the autumn season in your body. This is a time to turn inward, reflect, and gain clarity. It's also a time to prep for "winter" and accomplish those things that you've been putting off all month. You may feel inclined to finish projects, clean out your closet, meal prep, or deep clean the house. This is all thanks to progesterone, the calming, anti-anxiety hormone that regulates your mood and promotes deep sleep.

The thing is, in order to make progesterone, you must ovulate. After ovulation, the corpus luteum (what's left of the follicle after the egg was released) forms into an endocrine gland and starts making progesterone. This is meant to maintain and nourish a pregnancy, should a fertilized egg be implanted. If not, the corpus luteum gets reabsorbed, progesterone plummets, and you get your period! It's an AMAZING process.

The luteal phase is also when PMS may strike. The hormonal fluctuations may make your skin break out. Lower estrogen levels also mean less collagen, so your skin may feel less plump or radiant. Understanding why you're having certain symptoms at certain times will empower you to combat them in healthy ways. This is the magic of cycle tracking!

why keep track?

Tracking allows us to view our cycles in a unique way by examining the specifics and also taking a step back to observe overall themes. When we are deeply connected to what is going on inside our bodies, we begin to notice patterns in the way we feel or look that we may have otherwise written off as unimportant. One of the coolest things about cycle tracking is that it helps you connect the dots and prepare for what's ahead!

Let's say you felt really depressed or anxious in the few days leading up to your period last month. This month, you can mentally prepare by carving out some downtime. Or, maybe you had intense sugar cravings in your luteal phase. This month, you can get ready for that by balancing your blood sugar at every meal and having some healthier snack alternatives on hand. Ultimately, tracking provides a starting point for making better daily choices that accumulate over time.

On a basic level, tracking is incredibly helpful for knowing when your period will come and end, when you should use protection or avoid sex to prevent pregnancy, and for gaining a fundamental connection to your flow. And if you're trying to conceive, it's essential for fertility tracking.

On a deeper level, tracking can strengthen your body awareness (physically and emotionally) and connection to nature. Are you ovulating with the full moon or new moon? Do you sense the changing four seasons within your body each month? Do you notice how your emotions fluctuate? Once you become aware of these things, you realize that one, hormones are powerful influencers, and two, you don't have to be so hard on yourself. It's okay to feel super motivated and empowered one day and then have crappy days where you don't want to do anything. You can't be "on" every day of the month, just like the moon can't be full every day of the month. It's all part of your cyclical self!

All in all, by connecting to your cycle, you honor where you are in the present moment. Using this tracker will remind you to slow down, take a few moments for yourself, and reflect on your day, goals, worries, accomplishments, and more. This is a 90-day journal because after three months, you'll have a strong foundational knowledge of your personal cycle patterns. As I talk about in *The Happy Hormone Guide*, it takes three months to notice major cycle improvements after making changes to your nutrition and lifestyle. I created this journal to allow you to monitor that three-month journey. If you can track daily for 90 days, I promise you'll begin to really feel your flow and appreciate the power of your cycle.

what you'll track:

When I first started tracking, it was all about my period. Jotting down the day it started and ended was all I could handle. Once I got used to doing that, and started understanding its rhythm better, I felt comfortable tracking my ovulation using a thermometer or ovulation strips. That's when I really began noticing things on a deeper level—like how I feel a surge of energy and a happier mood before ovulation, only to feel it drop in the couple days post-ovulation. Or how hungry I am in the luteal phase and how I just want to organize everything in sight. Or how I feel deeply emotional and exhausted for two days before my period and yearn to hibernate and ponder life. As I slowly got in the habit of tracking my cycle, I learned so much about myself and my body. Over time, I began to understand how to better care for myself during each phase. This is my hope for you as you get started with The Happy Hormone Tracker. So, what will you be tracking exactly? Good question. I encourage you to start recording the following each day:

01. *cycle & moon phase*

Learning to understand which phase of your cycle you're in is the most important part of tracking. It provides a reference point for what to eat and how to live, work, and play. It allows you to work with your body and meet it where it's at.

02. *cervical mucus/bleeding*

Hormone levels fluctuate throughout your cycle and this influences changes to cervical mucus. Cervical mucus can fluctuate from crumbly and white to clear and stretchy. Tracking the consistency will help you gain a better understanding of where you are in your cycle. For instance, when you are at your most fertile, your mucus will have a stretchy, egg-white consistency. Your menstrual phase, on the other hand, is considered a "dry phase" for cervical mucus, even though you are bleeding. Day one of your menstrual phase begins on day one of heavy bleeding. During this time, it is important to monitor your flow, which should last anywhere from 3-7 days and start heavy before gradually tapering off. (If you experience spotting beforehand, this may be old blood from your last period.) There will be little to no cervical mucus for the first few days after your period as well. You'll feel dry until estrogen starts to rise, which can happen anywhere from day 6 to day 12.

03. *symptoms*

Hormonal fluctuations that are not in ideal ratios can sometimes present themselves through a range of symptoms—from fatigue to headaches to nausea. These experiences are clues to what is happening internally, possibly revealing an imbalance and something you should pay attention to rather than ignore or write off as "normal."

04. *ovarian pain*

If you experience sharp twinges on one or both sides of your abdomen, this can be a sign of mittelschmerz (sharp pain felt during ovulation when the egg ruptures from a follicle in one of your ovaries), or it can be linked to ovarian cysts. It's important to keep track of pain so you can report back to your health practitioner.

05. *basal body temp*

Basal body temperature is your body temperature at rest (right after you've woken up). This also fluctuates depending on when you are fertile. A definite sign that ovulation occurred is a rise in waking BBT for three consecutive days. Monitoring your BBT is one way to pinpoint if and when you ovulated. Purchase a basal body temp thermometer online or at a store like Target or CVS so you can begin to monitor your BBT.

06. *digestion*

Healthy digestion is essential for proper elimination of estrogen. Tracking allows you to recognize the foods that are helping move things along and making you feel good, as well as foods that often cause digestive upset, bloating, constipation, or other issues. If your digestion shifts in certain phases, you can eat to accommodate what's happening and be more aware of it in the next cycle. Elimination is KEY—so pay attention to it!

07. *mood*

Tracking changes in mood is important because it helps you prepare for what to expect in the next cycle. That way, if you know you get an energy crash and feel sad right after ovulation, you can be ready for it next time and give yourself the space to rest. Drastic mood changes can also be signs of hormone imbalance, imbalanced blood sugar, or nutrient deficiency. Our mood is often a direct reflection of what's happening in our bodies.

08. **stress level**

Stress is bad news for happy hormones. It signals your body to produce cortisol, your main fight-or-flight steroid hormone. Continuously high levels of cortisol can majorly impact hormone ratios. It's important to track stress levels so you can understand where added stress is stemming from in your life and make changes to address it.

09. **sex/libido**

It's normal for your libido to fluctuate throughout the month (it's highest around ovulation), but it's also something to be aware of and track. For instance, if you notice that it's totally nonexistent, it may be a sign that you have an imbalance.

10. **sleep**

Are you experiencing insomnia in a certain phase? Are you sleeping like a baby during another time in your cycle? These are important things to note. Proper sleep is one of the essential elements for hormone balance. Sleep issues can provide clues that you either need a lifestyle change or have an imbalance.

11. **supplements**

I recommend B vitamins, magnesium glycinate, vitamin D, zinc, iron, iodine and selenium, a daily probiotic, and algae-derived DHA/EPA for natural hormone balance, but you should consult your doctor or naturopath before starting supplementation. Then, use this tracker to monitor how your body reacts to them.

12. *food/cravings*

Look to the food charts in this book for plant-based recommendations on the best fuel for your body during each phase. There are four charts, one for each phase, that list out the specific macro and micronutrients your body needs at that time. Cravings often stem from imbalanced blood sugar or micronutrient deficiencies. Pay attention to when they happen and what you ate beforehand that may have triggered the craving. Or, if your cravings are more consistent, it might be worth asking your healthcare practitioner to perform a nutrient level test for more insight.

13. **exercise/movement**

The type of exercise you feel like doing will fluctuate throughout the month as well, so it can be fun to track what types of workouts you are drawn to, and when. Use the exercise chart on the next page as a guide. Daily movement is associated with better moods, lowered inflammation, and increased insulin sensitivity. It doesn't have to be a strenuous workout to be a good one!

14. **workflow/motivation**

This is a fun one to track because what you feel like working on may shift throughout your cycle. You may prefer creative work over detail-oriented work at different times. When you plan your work schedule around your cycle, you'll be able to work smarter!

~~~~~~~~~~

At the end of each week in this journal, you'll find a Weekly Reflection. This encourages you to take a moment to look back on the week and analyze what worked and what didn't, and also consider how you can improve or change things up for the week ahead. Reflecting on your week as a whole will also help you notice patterns that may be helping or harming your daily life and how you feel overall. It's also nice to look back on all that you have accomplished and the new ways you've learned to listen to your body!

exercise chart:

EXERCISES FOR EACH PHASE OF YOUR CYCLE

MENSTRUAL:
Soothing & Restorative Activities

- ☐ Yoga
- ☐ Pilates
- ☐ Walking
- ☐ Stretching
- ☐ Twisting

follicular:
Active/Cardio-Based Workouts

- ☐ Dance
- ☐ Biking
- ☐ Hiking
- ☐ Group Fitness
- ☐ Fast-Sequence Yoga

ovulation:
High-Impact Workouts

HIIT (HIGH-INTENSITY INTERVAL TRAINING)
SPIN CLASSES
BOOT CAMP
KICKBOXING
HOT YOGA
CIRCUIT TRAINING

luteal:

Core-Focused & Body Resistance

- ☐ Strength Training
- ☐ Mat Work
- ☐ Walking
- ☐ Pilates
- ☐ Yoga
- ☐ Elliptical

winter food chart:

VEGETABLES

beets
dulse
hijiki
kale
kelp
kombu
mushrooms (any variety)
nori
wakame
water chestnut

GRAINS

black rice
brown rice
buckwheat or kasha
wild rice

NUTS & SEEDS

chestnut
ground flaxseed
hazelnut
pumpkin seed

OTHER

bancha tea
coconut water
fennel tea
lemon water
licorice tea
liquid aminos
miso (organic)
sea salt
tamari (low sodium)
chlorella/liquid chlorophyll

LEGUMES

adzuki beans
black beans
edamame* (organic)
kidney beans
natto
tempeh* (organic)
tofu* (organic)

FRUITS

blackberries
blueberries
cranberries
grapes
watermelon

*Tempeh, tofu, and edamame are soy products that must be purchased organic, otherwise they are likely to be GMO.

spring food chart:

VEGETABLES

artichokes
asparagus
basil
broccoli
carrots
green beans
green peas
lettuce (Romaine, Bibb, Boston)
parsley
snow peas
sprouts (alfalfa, kale, broccoli, etc.)
sugar snap peas
zucchini

GRAINS

amaranth
barley (contains gluten)
farro (contains gluten)
oats (look for a gluten-free variety)
teff
quinoa

NUTS & SEEDS

brazil nuts
cashews (cashew butter)
flaxseeds (ground)
macadamia nuts
pumpkin/pepita seeds

OTHER

dairy-free yogurt, unsweetened
(coconut, almond, or cashew)
goji berries
capers
olives
pickles
pickled veggies
raw sauerkraut
vinegar *(apple cider, balsamic,
champagne, coconut, red wine, etc.)*

FRUITS

avocados
grapefruit
cherries
clementines
lemons
limes
lychees
mandarins (not canned)
nectarines
oranges
plums
pomegranates

LEGUMES

black-eyed peas	mung beans	* Tempeh, tofu, and edamame are soy
edamame*	split peas	products that must be purchased
lentils (any variety)	tempeh*	organic, otherwise they are likely
lima beans	tofu*	GMO products.

summer food chart:

GRAINS

amaranth
corn
quinoa

NUTS & SEEDS

almonds (almond butter)
pecans
pistachios
sesame seeds (tahini)
sunflower seeds (sunflower seed butter)

FRUITS

apricots
cantaloupes
clementines
coconuts
figs
guava
kiwi
mangoes
melons
papayas
passion fruit
pineapple
raspberries
strawberries

VEGETABLES

arugula
bell peppers
chard
chives
cucumbers
dandelion greens
eggplants
endive
fennel
okra
scallions
spinach
tomatoes

LEGUMES

mung beans
lentils (any variety)
split peas

OTHER

chicory
dandelion tea
turmeric

autumn food chart:

VEGETABLES

brussels sprouts
cabbage
cauliflower
celery
cilantro
collard greens
cucumber
daikon
garlic
ginger
jicama
leeks
mustard greens
onion
parsnips
pumpkin
radishes
rutabagas
shallots
squash (all varieties)
sweet potatoes
watercress
yams

GRAINS

brown rice
millet

NUTS & SEEDS

hickory
peanut (peanut butter)
pine nuts
sesame seeds (tahini)
sunflower seeds (sunflower seed butter)
walnuts

LEGUMES

chickpeas (garbanzo beans)
cannellini beans
great northern beans
navy beans

FRUITS

apples
bananas
dates
jackfruits
peaches
pears
persimmons
raisins

OTHER

cacao (raw/powdered form)
cinnamon
dandelion tea
fennel tea
licorice tea
mint
peppermint tea
spirulina

month: ....

DAY/	CYCLE DAY/

CYCLE PHASE:

- ☐ Menstrual
- ☐ Follicular
- ☐ Ovulatory
- ☐ Luteal

MOON PHASE:

Cervical Mucus:
check 'yes' or 'no' in boxes below   (yes) (no)

	yes	no
Tacky		
Crumbly		
Rubbery		
Creamy		
White		
Slippery		
Stringy		
Stretchy (highly fertile)		
Dry		

Bleeding/Spotting

none ☐ light ☐ medium ☐ heavy ☐

symptoms

- ☐ Cramps/Aches & Pains
- ☐ Headaches/Brain fog
- ☐ Lack of concentration
- ☐ Breast tenderness
- ☐ Nausea
- ☐ Loss of appetite
- ☐ Fatigue
- ☐ Insomnia
- ☐ Other:

ovulation?
☐ Yes   ☐ No

OVARIAN PAIN/CYSTS(which side?):

_____

BASAL BODY TEMPERATURE:

_____

Digestion:

☐ Regular ☐ Bloated ☐ Constipated ☐ Gassy

overall mood:

| happy | energetic | well-rested | calm | sad |

| irritable | depressed | anxious | wired | tired |

STRESS LEVEL/	low	medium	high
SEX or LIBIDO/	low	medium	high

SLEEP QUALITY	**SUPPLEMENTS:**

Nourishing Foods: _____

_____

Cravings: _____

_____

Exercise/Movement: _____

_____

_____

Workflow/Motivation: _____

_____

_____

month: ....

DAY/	CYCLE DAY/

CYCLE PHASE:

- ☐ Menstrual
- ☐ Follicular
- ☐ Ovulatory
- ☐ Luteal

MOON PHASE:

Cervical Mucus:
check 'yes' or 'no' in boxes below

	yes	no
Tacky		
Crumbly		
Rubbery		
Creamy		
White		
Slippery		
Stringy		
Stretchy (highly fertile)		
Dry		

Bleeding/Spotting

none ☐ light ☐ medium ☐ heavy ☐

symptoms
....

- ☐ Cramps/Aches & Pains
- ☐ Headaches/Brain fog
- ☐ Lack of concentration
- ☐ Breast tenderness
- ☐ Nausea
- ☐ Loss of appetite
- ☐ Fatigue
- ☐ Insomnia
- ☐ Other:

ovulation?
☐ Yes ☐ No

OVARIAN PAIN/CYSTS(which side?):
_____

BASAL BODY TEMPERATURE:
_____

Digestion:

☐ Regular   ☐ Bloated   ☐ Constipated   ☐ Gassy

overall mood:

(happy)   (energetic)   (well-rested)   (calm)   (sad)

(irritable)   (depressed)   (anxious)   (wired)   (tired)

STRESS LEVEL/	low	medium	high
SEX or LIBIDO/	low	medium	high

SLEEP QUALITY	SUPPLEMENTS:

Nourishing Foods: _____

Cravings: _____

Exercise/Movement: _____

Workflow/Motivation: _____

month: ....

DAY/	CYCLE DAY/

CYCLE PHASE:

- ☐ Menstrual
- ☐ Follicular
- ☐ Ovulatory
- ☐ Luteal

MOON PHASE:

Cervical Mucus: (yes) (no)
check 'yes' or 'no' in boxes below

	yes	no
Tacky		
Crumbly		
Rubbery		
Creamy		
White		
Slippery		
Stringy		
Stretchy (highly fertile)		
Dry		

Bleeding/Spotting

none ☐ light ☐ medium ☐ heavy ☐

symptoms
....

- ☐ Cramps/Aches & Pains
- ☐ Headaches/Brain fog
- ☐ Lack of concentration
- ☐ Breast tenderness
- ☐ Nausea
- ☐ Loss of appetite
- ☐ Fatigue
- ☐ Insomnia
- ☐ Other:

ovulation?

☐ Yes   ☐ No

OVARIAN PAIN/CYSTS(which side?):

_____

BASAL BODY TEMPERATURE:

_____

☐ Regular   ☐ Bloated   ☐ Constipated   ☐ Gassy

overall mood:

(happy)   (energetic)   (well-rested)   (calm)   (sad)

(irritable)   (depressed)   (anxious)   (wired)   (tired)

STRESS LEVEL/	low	medium	high
SEX or LIBIDO/	low	medium	high

SLEEP QUALITY	SUPPLEMENTS:

Nourishing Foods: _____

_____

Cravings: _____

_____

Exercise/Movement: _____

_____

_____

Workflow/Motivation: _____

_____

_____

month: ....

DAY/	CYCLE DAY/

CYCLE PHASE:

- ☐ Menstrual
- ☐ Follicular
- ☐ Ovulatory
- ☐ Luteal

MOON PHASE:

Cervical Mucus:
check 'yes' or 'no' in boxes below

(yes) (no)

	yes	no
Tacky		
Crumbly		
Rubbery		
Creamy		
White		
Slippery		
Stringy		
Stretchy (highly fertile)		
Dry		

Bleeding/Spotting

none ☐ light ☐ medium ☐ heavy ☐

symptoms
....

- ☐ Cramps/Aches & Pains
- ☐ Headaches/Brain fog
- ☐ Lack of concentration
- ☐ Breast tenderness
- ☐ Nausea
- ☐ Loss of appetite
- ☐ Fatigue
- ☐ Insomnia
- ☐ Other:

ovulation?
☐ Yes   ☐ No

OVARIAN PAIN/CYSTS(which side?):

_____

BASAL BODY TEMPERATURE:

_____

Digestion:

☐ Regular ☐ Bloated ☐ Constipated ☐ Gassy

overall mood:

(happy) (energetic) (well-rested) (calm) (sad)

(irritable) (depressed) (anxious) (wired) (tired)

STRESS LEVEL/	low	medium	high
SEX or LIBIDO/	low	medium	high

SLEEP QUALITY

SUPPLEMENTS:

Nourishing Foods: _____

Cravings: _____

Exercise/Movement: _____

Workflow/Motivation: _____

month: ....

DAY/	CYCLE DAY/

CYCLE PHASE:

- ☐ Menstrual
- ☐ Follicular
- ☐ Ovulatory
- ☐ Luteal

MOON PHASE:

Cervical Mucus: ⬭ yes   ⬭ no
check 'yes' or 'no' in boxes below

	yes	no
Tacky		
Crumbly		
Rubbery		
Creamy		
White		
Slippery		
Stringy		
Stretchy (highly fertile)		
Dry		

Bleeding/Spotting

none ☐   light ☐   medium ☐   heavy ☐

symptoms

....

- ☐ Cramps/Aches & Pains
- ☐ Headaches/Brain fog
- ☐ Lack of concentration
- ☐ Breast tenderness
- ☐ Nausea
- ☐ Loss of appetite
- ☐ Fatigue
- ☐ Insomnia
- ☐ Other:

ovulation?
☐ Yes   ☐ No

OVARIAN PAIN/CYSTS(which side?):

_____

BASAL BODY TEMPERATURE:

_____

☐ Regular ☐ Bloated ☐ Constipated ☐ Gassy

overall mood:

| happy | energetic | well-rested | calm | sad |

| irritable | depressed | anxious | wired | tired |

STRESS LEVEL/	low	medium	high
SEX or LIBIDO/	low	medium	high

SLEEP QUALITY	**SUPPLEMENTS:**

Nourishing Foods: _____

Cravings: _____

Exercise/Movement: _____

Workflow/Motivation: _____

month: ....

DAY/	CYCLE DAY/

CYCLE PHASE:

- ❑ Menstrual
- ❑ Follicular
- ❑ Ovulatory
- ❑ Luteal

MOON PHASE:

Cervical Mucus: (yes)   (no)
check 'yes' or 'no' in boxes below

	yes	no
Tacky		
Crumbly		
Rubbery		
Creamy		
White		
Slippery		
Stringy		
Stretchy (highly fertile)		
Dry		

Bleeding/Spotting

none ❑   light ❑   medium ❑   heavy ❑

symptoms
....

- ❑ Cramps/Aches & Pains
- ❑ Headaches/Brain fog
- ❑ Lack of concentration
- ❑ Breast tenderness
- ❑ Nausea
- ❑ Loss of appetite
- ❑ Fatigue
- ❑ Insomnia
- ❑ Other:

ovulation?

❑ Yes   ❑ No

OVARIAN PAIN/CYSTS(which side?):
_____

BASAL BODY TEMPERATURE:
_____

☐ Regular ☐ Bloated ☐ Constipated ☐ Gassy

overall mood:

happy	energetic	well-rested	calm	sad

irritable	depressed	anxious	wired	tired

STRESS LEVEL/	low	medium	high
SEX or LIBIDO/	low	medium	high

SLEEP QUALITY	SUPPLEMENTS:

Nourishing Foods: _____

_____

Cravings: _____

_____

Exercise/Movement: _____

_____

_____

Workflow/Motivation: _____

_____

_____

month: ....

DAY/	CYCLE DAY/

CYCLE PHASE:

- ☐ Menstrual
- ☐ Follicular
- ☐ Ovulatory
- ☐ Luteal

MOON PHASE:

Cervical Mucus:
check 'yes' or 'no' in boxes below   (yes)   (no)

	yes	no
Tacky		
Crumbly		
Rubbery		
Creamy		
White		
Slippery		
Stringy		
Stretchy (highly fertile)		
Dry		

Bleeding/Spotting

none ☐   light ☐   medium ☐   heavy ☐

symptoms
....

- ☐ Cramps/Aches & Pains
- ☐ Headaches/Brain fog
- ☐ Lack of concentration
- ☐ Breast tenderness
- ☐ Nausea
- ☐ Loss of appetite
- ☐ Fatigue
- ☐ Insomnia
- ☐ Other:

ovulation?
☐ Yes   ☐ No

OVARIAN PAIN/CYSTS(which side?):
_____

BASAL BODY TEMPERATURE:
_____

Digestion:

☐ Regular ☐ Bloated ☐ Constipated ☐ Gassy

overall mood:

(happy) (energetic) (well-rested) (calm) (sad)

(irritable) (depressed) (anxious) (wired) (tired)

STRESS LEVEL/	low	medium	high
SEX or LIBIDO/	low	medium	high

SLEEP QUALITY	SUPPLEMENTS:

Nourishing Foods: _____

_____

Cravings: _____

_____

Exercise/Movement: _____

_____

_____

Workflow/Motivation: _____

_____

_____

weekly reflection:

SKIN FLUCTUATIONS:

- ☐ Normal
- ☐ Oily
- ☐ Dry
- ☐ Blemishes
- ☐ Dull
- ☐ Glowy

Trying to drink more water? Meal plan? Limit social media?

. . .

Record your weekly habits here.

↓

Happy Weekly Habits: _____

_____

_____

_____

_____

_____

_____

What worked well this week?	*What did not work well this week?*

me time moments.

Record any special self-care practices like meditation, gratitude journaling, epsom salt bath, manicure... whatever "me time" means to you.

Me Time Moments: _____

_____

_____

_____

_____

_____

_____

_____

YOU GOT THIS

My most memorable moment of the week was . . .

_____

_____

_____

_____

_____

_____

_____

_____

_____

month: ....

DAY/	CYCLE DAY/

CYCLE PHASE:

- ☐ Menstrual
- ☐ Follicular
- ☐ Ovulatory
- ☐ Luteal

MOON PHASE:

Cervical Mucus:
check 'yes' or 'no' in boxes below

	yes	no
Tacky		
Crumbly		
Rubbery		
Creamy		
White		
Slippery		
Stringy		
Stretchy (highly fertile)		
Dry		

Bleeding/Spotting

none ☐　light ☐　medium ☐　heavy ☐

symptoms

....

- ☐ Cramps/Aches & Pains
- ☐ Headaches/Brain fog
- ☐ Lack of concentration
- ☐ Breast tenderness
- ☐ Nausea
- ☐ Loss of appetite
- ☐ Fatigue
- ☐ Insomnia
- ☐ Other:

ovulation?
☐ Yes　　☐ No

OVARIAN PAIN/CYSTS(which side?):

_____

BASAL BODY TEMPERATURE:

_____

Digestion:

☐ Regular   ☐ Bloated   ☐ Constipated   ☐ Gassy

overall mood:

(happy)   (energetic)   (well-rested)   (calm)   (sad)

(irritable)   (depressed)   (anxious)   (wired)   (tired)

STRESS LEVEL/	low	medium	high
SEX or LIBIDO/	low	medium	high

SLEEP QUALITY	SUPPLEMENTS:

Nourishing Foods: _____

Cravings: _____

Exercise/Movement: _____

Workflow/Motivation: _____

month: ....

DAY/	CYCLE DAY/

CYCLE PHASE:

- ❑ Menstrual
- ❑ Follicular
- ❑ Ovulatory
- ❑ Luteal

MOON PHASE:

Cervical Mucus:
check 'yes' or 'no' in boxes below

	yes	no
Tacky		
Crumbly		
Rubbery		
Creamy		
White		
Slippery		
Stringy		
Stretchy (highly fertile)		
Dry		

Bleeding/Spotting

none ❑   light ❑   medium ❑   heavy ❑

symptoms
....

- ❑ Cramps/Aches & Pains
- ❑ Headaches/Brain fog
- ❑ Lack of concentration
- ❑ Breast tenderness
- ❑ Nausea
- ❑ Loss of appetite
- ❑ Fatigue
- ❑ Insomnia
- ❑ Other:

ovulation?
❑ Yes   ❑ No

OVARIAN PAIN/CYSTS(which side?):
_____

BASAL BODY TEMPERATURE:
_____

☐ Regular   ☐ Bloated   ☐ Constipated   ☐ Gassy

overall mood:

(happy) (energetic) (well-rested) (calm) (sad)

(irritable) (depressed) (anxious) (wired) (tired)

STRESS LEVEL/	*low*	*medium*	*high*
SEX or LIBIDO/	*low*	*medium*	*high*

SLEEP QUALITY	SUPPLEMENTS:

Nourishing Foods: _____

_____

Cravings: _____

_____

Exercise/Movement: _____

_____

_____

Workflow/Motivation: _____

_____

_____

month: ....

DAY/	CYCLE DAY/

CYCLE PHASE:

- ❑ Menstrual
- ❑ Follicular
- ❑ Ovulatory
- ❑ Luteal

MOON PHASE:

Cervical Mucus:
check 'yes' or 'no' in boxes below

	yes	no
Tacky		
Crumbly		
Rubbery		
Creamy		
White		
Slippery		
Stringy		
Stretchy (highly fertile)		
Dry		

Bleeding/Spotting

none ❑ light ❑ medium ❑ heavy ❑

symptoms
....

- ❑ Cramps/Aches & Pains
- ❑ Headaches/Brain fog
- ❑ Lack of concentration
- ❑ Breast tenderness
- ❑ Nausea
- ❑ Loss of appetite
- ❑ Fatigue
- ❑ Insomnia
- ❑ Other:

ovulation?
❑ Yes   ❑ No

OVARIAN PAIN/CYSTS(which side?):
_____

BASAL BODY TEMPERATURE:
_____

Digestion:

☐ Regular ☐ Bloated ☐ Constipated ☐ Gassy

overall mood:

(happy) (energetic) (well-rested) (calm) (sad)

(irritable) (depressed) (anxious) (wired) (tired)

STRESS LEVEL/	low	medium	high
SEX or LIBIDO/	low	medium	high

SLEEP QUALITY	SUPPLEMENTS:

Nourishing Foods: _____

Cravings: _____

Exercise/Movement: _____

Workflow/Motivation: _____

month: ....

DAY/	CYCLE DAY/

CYCLE PHASE:

☐ Menstrual
☐ Follicular
☐ Ovulatory
☐ Luteal

MOON PHASE:

Cervical Mucus: (yes) (no)

check 'yes' or 'no' in boxes below

Tacky		
Crumbly		
Rubbery		
Creamy		
White		
Slippery		
Stringy		
Stretchy (highly fertile)		
Dry		

Bleeding/Spotting

none ☐ light ☐ medium ☐ heavy ☐

symptoms
....

☐ Cramps/Aches & Pains
☐ Headaches/Brain fog
☐ Lack of concentration
☐ Breast tenderness
☐ Nausea
☐ Loss of appetite
☐ Fatigue
☐ Insomnia
☐ Other:

ovulation?

☐ Yes   ☐ No

OVARIAN PAIN/CYSTS(which side?):
_____

BASAL BODY TEMPERATURE:
_____

Digestion:

☐ Regular ☐ Bloated ☐ Constipated ☐ Gassy

overall mood:

(happy) (energetic) (well-rested) (calm) (sad)

(irritable) (depressed) (anxious) (wired) (tired)

STRESS LEVEL/	low	medium	high
SEX or LIBIDO/	low	medium	high

SLEEP QUALITY	SUPPLEMENTS:

Nourishing Foods: _____

_____

Cravings: _____

_____

Exercise/Movement: _____

_____

_____

Workflow/Motivation: _____

_____

_____

month: ....

DAY/	CYCLE DAY/

CYCLE PHASE:

- ☐ Menstrual
- ☐ Follicular
- ☐ Ovulatory
- ☐ Luteal

MOON PHASE:

Cervical Mucus:
check 'yes' or 'no' in boxes below

	yes	no
Tacky		
Crumbly		
Rubbery		
Creamy		
White		
Slippery		
Stringy		
Stretchy (highly fertile)		
Dry		

Bleeding/Spotting

none ☐ light ☐ medium ☐ heavy ☐

symptoms
....

- ☐ Cramps/Aches & Pains
- ☐ Headaches/Brain fog
- ☐ Lack of concentration
- ☐ Breast tenderness
- ☐ Nausea
- ☐ Loss of appetite
- ☐ Fatigue
- ☐ Insomnia
- ☐ Other:

ovulation?
☐ Yes   ☐ No

OVARIAN PAIN/CYSTS(which side?):
_____

BASAL BODY TEMPERATURE:
_____

☐ Regular ☐ Bloated ☐ Constipated ☐ Gassy

overall mood:

happy	energetic	well-rested	calm	sad
irritable	depressed	anxious	wired	tired

STRESS LEVEL/	low	medium	high
SEX or LIBIDO/	low	medium	high

SLEEP QUALITY

SUPPLEMENTS:

Nourishing Foods: _____

_____

Cravings: _____

_____

Exercise/Movement: _____

_____

_____

Workflow/Motivation: _____

_____

_____

month: ....

DAY/	CYCLE DAY/

CYCLE PHASE:

- ☐ Menstrual
- ☐ Follicular
- ☐ Ovulatory
- ☐ Luteal

MOON PHASE:

Cervical Mucus: ⬭ yes ⬭ no
check 'yes' or 'no' in boxes below

Tacky		
Crumbly		
Rubbery		
Creamy		
White		
Slippery		
Stringy		
Stretchy (highly fertile)		
Dry		

Bleeding/Spotting

none ☐ light ☐ medium ☐ heavy ☐

symptoms
....

- ☐ Cramps/Aches & Pains
- ☐ Headaches/Brain fog
- ☐ Lack of concentration
- ☐ Breast tenderness
- ☐ Nausea
- ☐ Loss of appetite
- ☐ Fatigue
- ☐ Insomnia
- ☐ Other:

ovulation?
☐ Yes   ☐ No

OVARIAN PAIN/CYSTS(which side?):
_____

BASAL BODY TEMPERATURE:
_____

Digestion:

☐ Regular ☐ Bloated ☐ Constipated ☐ Gassy

overall mood:

happy	energetic	well-rested	calm	sad
irritable	depressed	anxious	wired	tired

STRESS LEVEL/	*low*	*medium*	*high*
SEX or LIBIDO/	*low*	*medium*	*high*

SLEEP QUALITY

SUPPLEMENTS:

Nourishing Foods: _____

_____

Cravings: _____

_____

Exercise/Movement: _____

_____

_____

Workflow/Motivation: _____

_____

_____

month: ....

DAY/	CYCLE DAY/

CYCLE PHASE:	MOON PHASE:

CYCLE PHASE:

- ☐ Menstrual
- ☐ Follicular
- ☐ Ovulatory
- ☐ Luteal

MOON PHASE:

Cervical Mucus:
check 'yes' or 'no' in boxes below

(yes) (no)

	yes	no
Tacky		
Crumbly		
Rubbery		
Creamy		
White		
Slippery		
Stringy		
Stretchy (highly fertile)		
Dry		

Bleeding/Spotting

none ☐ light ☐ medium ☐ heavy ☐

symptoms
....

- ☐ Cramps/Aches & Pains
- ☐ Headaches/Brain fog
- ☐ Lack of concentration
- ☐ Breast tenderness
- ☐ Nausea
- ☐ Loss of appetite
- ☐ Fatigue
- ☐ Insomnia
- ☐ Other:

ovulation?
☐ Yes   ☐ No

OVARIAN PAIN/CYSTS(which side?):
_____

BASAL BODY TEMPERATURE:
_____

Digestion:

☐ Regular ☐ Bloated ☐ Constipated ☐ Gassy

overall mood:

(happy) (energetic) (well-rested) (calm) (sad)

(irritable) (depressed) (anxious) (wired) (tired)

STRESS LEVEL/	low	medium	high
SEX or LIBIDO/	low	medium	high

SLEEP QUALITY	SUPPLEMENTS:

Nourishing Foods: _____

_____

Cravings: _____

_____

Exercise/Movement: _____

_____

Workflow/Motivation: _____

_____

_____

weekly reflection:

....

SKIN FLUCTUATIONS:

- ☐ Normal
- ☐ Oily
- ☐ Dry
- ☐ Blemishes
- ☐ Dull
- ☐ Glowy

Trying to drink more water? Meal plan? Limit social media?

. . .

Record your weekly habits here.

↓

Happy Weekly Habits: _____

_____

_____

_____

_____

_____

_____

What worked well this week?	*What did not work well this week?*

me time moments.

Record any special self-care practices like meditation, gratitude journaling, epsom salt bath, manicure... whatever "me time" means to you.

Me Time Moments: _____

_____

_____

_____

_____

_____

_____

_____

YOU GOT THIS

My most memorable moment of the week was . . .

_____

_____

_____

_____

_____

_____

_____

_____

month: ....

DAY/	CYCLE DAY/

CYCLE PHASE:	MOON PHASE:

CYCLE PHASE:

- ☐ Menstrual
- ☐ Follicular
- ☐ Ovulatory
- ☐ Luteal

MOON PHASE:

Cervical Mucus: ⬭ yes ⬭ no
check 'yes' or 'no' in boxes below

	yes	no
Tacky		
Crumbly		
Rubbery		
Creamy		
White		
Slippery		
Stringy		
Stretchy (highly fertile)		
Dry		

Bleeding/Spotting

none ☐ light ☐ medium ☐ heavy ☐

symptoms
....

- ☐ Cramps/Aches & Pains
- ☐ Headaches/Brain fog
- ☐ Lack of concentration
- ☐ Breast tenderness
- ☐ Nausea
- ☐ Loss of appetite
- ☐ Fatigue
- ☐ Insomnia
- ☐ Other:

ovulation?
☐ Yes   ☐ No

OVARIAN PAIN/CYSTS(which side?):
_____

BASAL BODY TEMPERATURE:
_____

Digestion:

☐ Regular ☐ Bloated ☐ Constipated ☐ Gassy

overall mood:

(happy) (energetic) (well-rested) (calm) (sad)

(irritable) (depressed) (anxious) (wired) (tired)

STRESS LEVEL/	low	medium	high
SEX or LIBIDO/	low	medium	high

SLEEP QUALITY	SUPPLEMENTS:

Nourishing Foods: _____

_____

Cravings: _____

_____

Exercise/Movement: _____

_____

_____

Workflow/Motivation: _____

_____

_____

month: ....

DAY/	CYCLE DAY/

CYCLE PHASE:	MOON PHASE:

CYCLE PHASE:

☐ Menstrual
☐ Follicular
☐ Ovulatory
☐ Luteal

MOON PHASE:

Cervical Mucus: ⬭ yes ⬭ no
check 'yes' or 'no' in boxes below

	yes	no
Tacky		
Crumbly		
Rubbery		
Creamy		
White		
Slippery		
Stringy		
Stretchy (highly fertile)		
Dry		

Bleeding/Spotting

none ☐ light ☐ medium ☐ heavy ☐

symptoms
....

☐ Cramps/Aches & Pains
☐ Headaches/Brain fog
☐ Lack of concentration
☐ Breast tenderness
☐ Nausea
☐ Loss of appetite
☐ Fatigue
☐ Insomnia
☐ Other:

ovulation?
☐ Yes ☐ No

OVARIAN PAIN/CYSTS(which side?):
_____

BASAL BODY TEMPERATURE:
_____

Digestion:

☐ Regular ☐ Bloated ☐ Constipated ☐ Gassy

overall mood:

(happy) (energetic) (well-rested) (calm) (sad)

(irritable) (depressed) (anxious) (wired) (tired)

STRESS LEVEL/	low	medium	high
SEX or LIBIDO/	low	medium	high

SLEEP QUALITY	**SUPPLEMENTS:**

Nourishing Foods: _____

_____

Cravings: _____

_____

Exercise/Movement: _____

_____

_____

Workflow/Motivation: _____

_____

_____

month: ....

DAY/	CYCLE DAY/

CYCLE PHASE:

- ☐ Menstrual
- ☐ Follicular
- ☐ Ovulatory
- ☐ Luteal

MOON PHASE:

Cervical Mucus:

❨ yes ❩ ❨ no ❩

check 'yes' or 'no' in boxes below

	yes	no
Tacky		
Crumbly		
Rubbery		
Creamy		
White		
Slippery		
Stringy		
Stretchy (highly fertile)		
Dry		

Bleeding/Spotting

none ☐ light ☐ medium ☐ heavy ☐

symptoms
....

- ☐ Cramps/Aches & Pains
- ☐ Headaches/Brain fog
- ☐ Lack of concentration
- ☐ Breast tenderness
- ☐ Nausea
- ☐ Loss of appetite
- ☐ Fatigue
- ☐ Insomnia
- ☐ Other:

ovulation?

☐ Yes   ☐ No

OVARIAN PAIN/CYSTS(which side?):

_____

BASAL BODY TEMPERATURE:

_____

Digestion:

☐ Regular ☐ Bloated ☐ Constipated ☐ Gassy

overall mood:

(happy) (energetic) (well-rested) (calm) (sad)

(irritable) (depressed) (anxious) (wired) (tired)

STRESS LEVEL/	low	medium	high
SEX or LIBIDO/	low	medium	high

SLEEP QUALITY

SUPPLEMENTS:

Nourishing Foods: _____

Cravings: _____

Exercise/Movement: _____

Workflow/Motivation: _____

month: ....

DAY/	CYCLE DAY/

CYCLE PHASE:

- ❑ Menstrual
- ❑ Follicular
- ❑ Ovulatory
- ❑ Luteal

MOON PHASE:

Cervical Mucus:
check 'yes' or 'no' in boxes below

	yes	no
Tacky		
Crumbly		
Rubbery		
Creamy		
White		
Slippery		
Stringy		
Stretchy (highly fertile)		
Dry		

Bleeding/Spotting

none ❑   light ❑   medium ❑   heavy ❑

symptoms
....

- ❑ Cramps/Aches & Pains
- ❑ Headaches/Brain fog
- ❑ Lack of concentration
- ❑ Breast tenderness
- ❑ Nausea
- ❑ Loss of appetite
- ❑ Fatigue
- ❑ Insomnia
- ❑ Other:

ovulation?
❑ Yes   ❑ No

OVARIAN PAIN/CYSTS(which side?):

BASAL BODY TEMPERATURE:

Digestion:

☐ Regular ☐ Bloated ☐ Constipated ☐ Gassy

overall mood:

(happy) (energetic) (well-rested) (calm) (sad)

(irritable) (depressed) (anxious) (wired) (tired)

STRESS LEVEL/	low	medium	high
SEX or LIBIDO/	low	medium	high

SLEEP QUALITY	SUPPLEMENTS:

Nourishing Foods: _____

_____

Cravings: _____

_____

Exercise/Movement: _____

_____

_____

Workflow/Motivation: _____

_____

_____

month: ....

CYCLE PHASE:

- ☐ Menstrual
- ☐ Follicular
- ☐ Ovulatory
- ☐ Luteal

MOON PHASE:

Cervical Mucus:
check 'yes' or 'no' in boxes below   (yes) (no)

	yes	no
Tacky		
Crumbly		
Rubbery		
Creamy		
White		
Slippery		
Stringy		
Stretchy (highly fertile)		
Dry		

Bleeding/Spotting

none ☐ light ☐ medium ☐ heavy ☐

symptoms
....

- ☐ Cramps/Aches & Pains
- ☐ Headaches/Brain fog
- ☐ Lack of concentration
- ☐ Breast tenderness
- ☐ Nausea
- ☐ Loss of appetite
- ☐ Fatigue
- ☐ Insomnia
- ☐ Other:

ovulation?
☐ Yes   ☐ No

OVARIAN PAIN/CYSTS(which side?):
_____

BASAL BODY TEMPERATURE:
_____

☐ Regular ☐ Bloated ☐ Constipated ☐ Gassy

overall mood:

happy	energetic	well-rested	calm	sad

irritable	depressed	anxious	wired	tired

STRESS LEVEL/	*low*	*medium*	*high*	
SEX or LIBIDO/	*low*	*medium*	*high*	

SLEEP QUALITY	SUPPLEMENTS:

Nourishing Foods: _____

Cravings: _____

Exercise/Movement: _____

Workflow/Motivation: _____

month: ....

DAY/	CYCLE DAY/

CYCLE PHASE:

- ☐ Menstrual
- ☐ Follicular
- ☐ Ovulatory
- ☐ Luteal

MOON PHASE:

Cervical Mucus:
check 'yes' or 'no' in boxes below   ⬭ yes ⬭ no

	yes	no
Tacky		
Crumbly		
Rubbery		
Creamy		
White		
Slippery		
Stringy		
Stretchy (highly fertile)		
Dry		

Bleeding/Spotting

none ☐ light ☐ medium ☐ heavy ☐

symptoms
....

- ☐ Cramps/Aches & Pains
- ☐ Headaches/Brain fog
- ☐ Lack of concentration
- ☐ Breast tenderness
- ☐ Nausea
- ☐ Loss of appetite
- ☐ Fatigue
- ☐ Insomnia
- ☐ Other:

ovulation?
☐ Yes   ☐ No

OVARIAN PAIN/CYSTS(which side?):
_____

BASAL BODY TEMPERATURE:
_____

☐ Regular ☐ Bloated ☐ Constipated ☐ Gassy

overall mood:

(happy) (energetic) (well-rested) (calm) (sad)

(irritable) (depressed) (anxious) (wired) (tired)

STRESS LEVEL/	low	medium	high
SEX or LIBIDO/	low	medium	high

SLEEP QUALITY	**SUPPLEMENTS:**

Nourishing Foods: _____

_____

Cravings: _____

_____

Exercise/Movement: _____

_____

_____

Workflow/Motivation: _____

_____

_____

month: ....

DAY/	CYCLE DAY/

CYCLE PHASE:

- ☐ Menstrual
- ☐ Follicular
- ☐ Ovulatory
- ☐ Luteal

MOON PHASE:

Cervical Mucus:
check 'yes' or 'no' in boxes below   (yes) (no)

Tacky		
Crumbly		
Rubbery		
Creamy		
White		
Slippery		
Stringy		
Stretchy (highly fertile)		
Dry		

Bleeding/Spotting

none ☐ light ☐ medium ☐ heavy ☐

symptoms
....

- ☐ Cramps/Aches & Pains
- ☐ Headaches/Brain fog
- ☐ Lack of concentration
- ☐ Breast tenderness
- ☐ Nausea
- ☐ Loss of appetite
- ☐ Fatigue
- ☐ Insomnia
- ☐ Other:

ovulation?
☐ Yes   ☐ No

OVARIAN PAIN/CYSTS(which side?):

_____

BASAL BODY TEMPERATURE:

_____

Digestion:

☐ Regular ☐ Bloated ☐ Constipated ☐ Gassy

overall mood:

(happy) (energetic) (well-rested) (calm) (sad)

(irritable) (depressed) (anxious) (wired) (tired)

STRESS LEVEL/	low	medium	high
SEX or LIBIDO/	low	medium	high

SLEEP QUALITY	SUPPLEMENTS:

Nourishing Foods: _____

_____

Cravings: _____

_____

Exercise/Movement: _____

_____

_____

Workflow/Motivation: _____

_____

_____

weekly reflection:

....

SKIN FLUCTUATIONS:

☐ Normal

☐ Oily

☐ Dry

☐ Blemishes

☐ Dull

☐ Glowy

Trying to drink more water? Meal plan? Limit social media?

. . .

Record your weekly habits here.

↓

Happy Weekly Habits: _____

_____

_____

_____

_____

_____

_____

What worked well this week?	*What did not work well this week?*
....	....

me time moments.

Record any special self-care practices like meditation,
gratitude journaling, epsom salt bath, manicure...
whatever "me time" means to you.

Me Time Moments: _____

_____

_____

_____

_____

_____

_____

_____

YOU
GOT
THIS

My most memorable moment of the week was . . .

_____

_____

_____

_____

_____

_____

_____

month: ....

DAY/	CYCLE DAY/

CYCLE PHASE:

- ❑ Menstrual
- ❑ Follicular
- ❑ Ovulatory
- ❑ Luteal

MOON PHASE:

Cervical Mucus: ⬭yes ⬭no
check 'yes' or 'no' in boxes below

Tacky		
Crumbly		
Rubbery		
Creamy		
White		
Slippery		
Stringy		
Stretchy (highly fertile)		
Dry		

Bleeding/Spotting

none ❑ light ❑ medium ❑ heavy ❑

symptoms

....

- ❑ Cramps/Aches & Pains
- ❑ Headaches/Brain fog
- ❑ Lack of concentration
- ❑ Breast tenderness
- ❑ Nausea
- ❑ Loss of appetite
- ❑ Fatigue
- ❑ Insomnia
- ❑ Other:

ovulation?
❑ Yes ❑ No

OVARIAN PAIN/CYSTS(which side?):

BASAL BODY TEMPERATURE:

☐ Regular ☐ Bloated ☐ Constipated ☐ Gassy

overall mood:

(happy) (energetic) (well-rested) (calm) (sad)

(irritable) (depressed) (anxious) (wired) (tired)

STRESS LEVEL/	low	medium	high
SEX or LIBIDO/	low	medium	high

SLEEP QUALITY	SUPPLEMENTS:

Nourishing Foods: _____

_____

Cravings: _____

_____

Exercise/Movement: _____

_____

_____

Workflow/Motivation: _____

_____

_____

month:

CYCLE PHASE:

- ☐ Menstrual
- ☐ Follicular
- ☐ Ovulatory
- ☐ Luteal

MOON PHASE:

Cervical Mucus:
check 'yes' or 'no' in boxes below

(yes) (no)

	yes	no
Tacky		
Crumbly		
Rubbery		
Creamy		
White		
Slippery		
Stringy		
Stretchy (highly fertile)		
Dry		

Bleeding/Spotting

none ☐ light ☐ medium ☐ heavy ☐

symptoms

- ☐ Cramps/Aches & Pains
- ☐ Headaches/Brain fog
- ☐ Lack of concentration
- ☐ Breast tenderness
- ☐ Nausea
- ☐ Loss of appetite
- ☐ Fatigue
- ☐ Insomnia
- ☐ Other:

ovulation?

☐ Yes   ☐ No

OVARIAN PAIN/CYSTS(which side?):

BASAL BODY TEMPERATURE:

☐ Regular   ☐ Bloated   ☐ Constipated   ☐ Gassy

overall mood:

happy	energetic	well-rested	calm	sad
irritable	depressed	anxious	wired	tired

STRESS LEVEL/	low	medium	high
SEX or LIBIDO/	low	medium	high

SLEEP QUALITY	SUPPLEMENTS:

Nourishing Foods: _____

_____

Cravings: _____

_____

Exercise/Movement: _____

_____

_____

Workflow/Motivation: _____

_____

_____

month: ....

DAY/	CYCLE DAY/

CYCLE PHASE:

- ☐ Menstrual
- ☐ Follicular
- ☐ Ovulatory
- ☐ Luteal

MOON PHASE:

Cervical Mucus: ⬭ yes ⬭ no
check 'yes' or 'no' in boxes below

	yes	no
Tacky		
Crumbly		
Rubbery		
Creamy		
White		
Slippery		
Stringy		
Stretchy (highly fertile)		
Dry		

Bleeding/Spotting

none ☐ light ☐ medium ☐ heavy ☐

symptoms
....

- ☐ Cramps/Aches & Pains
- ☐ Headaches/Brain fog
- ☐ Lack of concentration
- ☐ Breast tenderness
- ☐ Nausea
- ☐ Loss of appetite
- ☐ Fatigue
- ☐ Insomnia
- ☐ Other:

ovulation?
☐ Yes ☐ No

OVARIAN PAIN/CYSTS(which side?):
_____

BASAL BODY TEMPERATURE:
_____

☐ Regular ☐ Bloated ☐ Constipated ☐ Gassy

overall mood:

happy	energetic	well-rested	calm	sad
irritable	depressed	anxious	wired	tired

STRESS LEVEL/	low	medium	high
SEX or LIBIDO/	low	medium	high

SLEEP QUALITY	**SUPPLEMENTS:**

Nourishing Foods: _____

_____

Cravings: _____

_____

Exercise/Movement: _____

_____

_____

Workflow/Motivation: _____

_____

_____

month: ....

DAY/	CYCLE DAY/

CYCLE PHASE:

- ☐ Menstrual
- ☐ Follicular
- ☐ Ovulatory
- ☐ Luteal

MOON PHASE:

Cervical Mucus:
check 'yes' or 'no' in boxes below

	yes	no
Tacky		
Crumbly		
Rubbery		
Creamy		
White		
Slippery		
Stringy		
Stretchy (highly fertile)		
Dry		

Bleeding/Spotting

none ☐ light ☐ medium ☐ heavy ☐

symptoms
....

- ☐ Cramps/Aches & Pains
- ☐ Headaches/Brain fog
- ☐ Lack of concentration
- ☐ Breast tenderness
- ☐ Nausea
- ☐ Loss of appetite
- ☐ Fatigue
- ☐ Insomnia
- ☐ Other:

ovulation?
☐ Yes   ☐ No

OVARIAN PAIN/CYSTS(which side?):
_____

BASAL BODY TEMPERATURE:
_____

☐ Regular ☐ Bloated ☐ Constipated ☐ Gassy

overall mood:

(happy) (energetic) (well-rested) (calm) (sad)

(irritable) (depressed) (anxious) (wired) (tired)

STRESS LEVEL/	low	medium	high
SEX or LIBIDO/	low	medium	high

SLEEP QUALITY

SUPPLEMENTS:

Nourishing Foods: _____

_____

Cravings: _____

_____

Exercise/Movement: _____

_____

_____

Workflow/Motivation: _____

_____

_____

month: ....

DAY/	CYCLE DAY/

CYCLE PHASE:

- ❑ Menstrual
- ❑ Follicular
- ❑ Ovulatory
- ❑ Luteal

MOON PHASE:

Cervical Mucus: (yes) (no)
check 'yes' or 'no' in boxes below

	yes	no
Tacky		
Crumbly		
Rubbery		
Creamy		
White		
Slippery		
Stringy		
Stretchy (highly fertile)		
Dry		

Bleeding/Spotting

none ❑   light ❑   medium ❑   heavy ❑

symptoms
....

- ❑ Cramps/Aches & Pains
- ❑ Headaches/Brain fog
- ❑ Lack of concentration
- ❑ Breast tenderness
- ❑ Nausea
- ❑ Loss of appetite
- ❑ Fatigue
- ❑ Insomnia
- ❑ Other:

ovulation?
❑ Yes   ❑ No

OVARIAN PAIN/CYSTS(which side?):

_____

BASAL BODY TEMPERATURE:

_____

Digestion:

☐ Regular   ☐ Bloated   ☐ Constipated   ☐ Gassy

overall mood:

(happy)   (energetic)   (well-rested)   (calm)   (sad)

(irritable)   (depressed)   (anxious)   (wired)   (tired)

STRESS LEVEL/	low	medium	high
SEX or LIBIDO/	low	medium	high

SLEEP QUALITY	SUPPLEMENTS:

Nourishing Foods: _____

_____

Cravings: _____

_____

Exercise/Movement: _____

_____

_____

Workflow/Motivation: _____

_____

_____

month: ....

DAY/	CYCLE DAY/

CYCLE PHASE:	**MOON PHASE:**

CYCLE PHASE:

- ❑ Menstrual
- ❑ Follicular
- ❑ Ovulatory
- ❑ Luteal

MOON PHASE:

Cervical Mucus: ⬭ yes   ⬭ no
check 'yes' or 'no' in boxes below

	yes	no
Tacky		
Crumbly		
Rubbery		
Creamy		
White		
Slippery		
Stringy		
Stretchy (highly fertile)		
Dry		

Bleeding/Spotting

none ❑   light ❑   medium ❑   heavy ❑

symptoms
....

- ❑ Cramps/Aches & Pains
- ❑ Headaches/Brain fog
- ❑ Lack of concentration
- ❑ Breast tenderness
- ❑ Nausea
- ❑ Loss of appetite
- ❑ Fatigue
- ❑ Insomnia
- ❑ Other:

ovulation?
❑ Yes   ❑ No

OVARIAN PAIN/CYSTS(which side?):
_____

BASAL BODY TEMPERATURE:
_____

Digestion:

☐ Regular ☐ Bloated ☐ Constipated ☐ Gassy

overall mood:

(happy) (energetic) (well-rested) (calm) (sad)

(irritable) (depressed) (anxious) (wired) (tired)

STRESS LEVEL/	low	medium	high
SEX or LIBIDO/	low	medium	high

SLEEP QUALITY	SUPPLEMENTS:

Nourishing Foods: _____

Cravings: _____

Exercise/Movement: _____

Workflow/Motivation: _____

month: ....

DAY/	CYCLE DAY/

CYCLE PHASE:

- ☐ Menstrual
- ☐ Follicular
- ☐ Ovulatory
- ☐ Luteal

MOON PHASE:

Cervical Mucus:
check 'yes' or 'no' in boxes below   (yes)   (no)

	yes	no
Tacky		
Crumbly		
Rubbery		
Creamy		
White		
Slippery		
Stringy		
Stretchy (highly fertile)		
Dry		

Bleeding/Spotting

none ☐   light ☐   medium ☐   heavy ☐

symptoms
....

- ☐ Cramps/Aches & Pains
- ☐ Headaches/Brain fog
- ☐ Lack of concentration
- ☐ Breast tenderness
- ☐ Nausea
- ☐ Loss of appetite
- ☐ Fatigue
- ☐ Insomnia
- ☐ Other:

ovulation?
☐ Yes   ☐ No

OVARIAN PAIN/CYSTS(which side?):

_____

BASAL BODY TEMPERATURE:

_____

Digestion:

☐ Regular ☐ Bloated ☐ Constipated ☐ Gassy

overall mood:

(happy) (energetic) (well-rested) (calm) (sad)

(irritable) (depressed) (anxious) (wired) (tired)

| STRESS LEVEL/ | low | medium | high |
| SEX or LIBIDO/ | low | medium | high |

SLEEP QUALITY

SUPPLEMENTS:

Nourishing Foods: _____

Cravings: _____

Exercise/Movement: _____

Workflow/Motivation: _____

weekly reflection:

SKIN FLUCTUATIONS:

- ☐ Normal
- ☐ Oily
- ☐ Dry
- ☐ Blemishes
- ☐ Dull
- ☐ Glowy

Trying to drink more water? Meal plan? Limit social media?

. . .

Record your weekly habits here.

↓

Happy Weekly Habits: _____

_____

_____

_____

_____

_____

_____

What worked well this week?	*What did not work well this week?*

me time moments.

Record any special self-care practices like meditation, gratitude journaling, epsom salt bath, manicure... whatever "me time" means to you.

Me Time Moments: _____

_____

_____

_____

_____

_____

_____

_____

YOU
GOT
THIS

My most memorable moment of the week was . . .

_____

_____

_____

_____

_____

_____

_____

_____

month: ....

DAY/	CYCLE DAY/

CYCLE PHASE:

☐ Menstrual
☐ Follicular
☐ Ovulatory
☐ Luteal

MOON PHASE:

Cervical Mucus: ⬭ yes   ⬭ no
check 'yes' or 'no' in boxes below

Tacky		
Crumbly		
Rubbery		
Creamy		
White		
Slippery		
Stringy		
Stretchy (highly fertile)		
Dry		

Bleeding/Spotting

none ☐ light ☐ medium ☐ heavy ☐

symptoms
....

☐ Cramps/Aches & Pains
☐ Headaches/Brain fog
☐ Lack of concentration
☐ Breast tenderness
☐ Nausea
☐ Loss of appetite
☐ Fatigue
☐ Insomnia
☐ Other:

ovulation?
☐ Yes   ☐ No

OVARIAN PAIN/CYSTS(which side?):
_____

BASAL BODY TEMPERATURE:
_____

☐ Regular ☐ Bloated ☐ Constipated ☐ Gassy

overall mood:

happy	energetic	well-rested	calm	sad

irritable	depressed	anxious	wired	tired

STRESS LEVEL/	low	medium	high
SEX or LIBIDO/	low	medium	high

SLEEP QUALITY	SUPPLEMENTS:

Nourishing Foods: _____

_____

Cravings: _____

_____

Exercise/Movement: _____

_____

_____

Workflow/Motivation: _____

_____

_____

month: ....

DAY/	CYCLE DAY/

CYCLE PHASE:

☐ Menstrual
☐ Follicular
☐ Ovulatory
☐ Luteal

MOON PHASE:

Cervical Mucus:
check 'yes' or 'no' in boxes below

⬭ yes ⬭ no

	yes	no
Tacky		
Crumbly		
Rubbery		
Creamy		
White		
Slippery		
Stringy		
Stretchy (highly fertile)		
Dry		

Bleeding/Spotting

none ☐ light ☐ medium ☐ heavy ☐

symptoms
....

☐ Cramps/Aches & Pains
☐ Headaches/Brain fog
☐ Lack of concentration
☐ Breast tenderness
☐ Nausea
☐ Loss of appetite
☐ Fatigue
☐ Insomnia
☐ Other:

ovulation?
☐ Yes ☐ No

OVARIAN PAIN/CYSTS(which side?):
_____

BASAL BODY TEMPERATURE:
_____

Digestion:

☐ Regular ☐ Bloated ☐ Constipated ☐ Gassy

overall mood:

(happy) (energetic) (well-rested) (calm) (sad)

(irritable) (depressed) (anxious) (wired) (tired)

STRESS LEVEL/	*low*	*medium*	*high*
SEX or LIBIDO/	*low*	*medium*	*high*

SLEEP QUALITY	**SUPPLEMENTS:**

Nourishing Foods: _____

_____

Cravings: _____

_____

Exercise/Movement: _____

_____

_____

Workflow/Motivation: _____

_____

_____

month: ....

DAY/	CYCLE DAY/

CYCLE PHASE:

- ☐ Menstrual
- ☐ Follicular
- ☐ Ovulatory
- ☐ Luteal

MOON PHASE:

Cervical Mucus:
check 'yes' or 'no' in boxes below   (yes) (no)

	yes	no
Tacky		
Crumbly		
Rubbery		
Creamy		
White		
Slippery		
Stringy		
Stretchy (highly fertile)		
Dry		

Bleeding/Spotting

none ☐   light ☐   medium ☐   heavy ☐

symptoms
....

- ☐ Cramps/Aches & Pains
- ☐ Headaches/Brain fog
- ☐ Lack of concentration
- ☐ Breast tenderness
- ☐ Nausea
- ☐ Loss of appetite
- ☐ Fatigue
- ☐ Insomnia
- ☐ Other:

ovulation?
☐ Yes   ☐ No

OVARIAN PAIN/CYSTS(which side?):
_____

BASAL BODY TEMPERATURE:
_____

Digestion:

☐ Regular   ☐ Bloated   ☐ Constipated   ☐ Gassy

overall mood:

(happy)   (energetic)   (well-rested)   (calm)   (sad)

(irritable)   (depressed)   (anxious)   (wired)   (tired)

STRESS LEVEL/	low	medium	high
SEX or LIBIDO/	low	medium	high

SLEEP QUALITY	SUPPLEMENTS:

Nourishing Foods: _____

_____

Cravings: _____

_____

Exercise/Movement: _____

_____

_____

Workflow/Motivation: _____

_____

_____

month: ....

DAY/	CYCLE DAY/

CYCLE PHASE:

- ☐ Menstrual
- ☐ Follicular
- ☐ Ovulatory
- ☐ Luteal

MOON PHASE:

Cervical Mucus:
check 'yes' or 'no' in boxes below   (yes) (no)

	yes	no
Tacky		
Crumbly		
Rubbery		
Creamy		
White		
Slippery		
Stringy		
Stretchy (highly fertile)		
Dry		

Bleeding/Spotting

none ☐ light ☐ medium ☐ heavy ☐

symptoms
....

- ☐ Cramps/Aches & Pains
- ☐ Headaches/Brain fog
- ☐ Lack of concentration
- ☐ Breast tenderness
- ☐ Nausea
- ☐ Loss of appetite
- ☐ Fatigue
- ☐ Insomnia
- ☐ Other:

ovulation?
☐ Yes   ☐ No

OVARIAN PAIN/CYSTS(which side?):
_____

BASAL BODY TEMPERATURE:
_____

☐ Regular   ☐ Bloated   ☐ Constipated   ☐ Gassy

overall mood:

(happy)   (energetic)   (well-rested)   (calm)   (sad)

(irritable)   (depressed)   (anxious)   (wired)   (tired)

STRESS LEVEL/	low	medium	high
SEX or LIBIDO/	low	medium	high

SLEEP QUALITY	**SUPPLEMENTS:**

Nourishing Foods: _____

Cravings: _____

Exercise/Movement: _____

Workflow/Motivation: _____

month: ....

DAY/	CYCLE DAY/

CYCLE PHASE:

- ☐ Menstrual
- ☐ Follicular
- ☐ Ovulatory
- ☐ Luteal

MOON PHASE:

Cervical Mucus: (yes) (no)
check 'yes' or 'no' in boxes below

	yes	no
Tacky		
Crumbly		
Rubbery		
Creamy		
White		
Slippery		
Stringy		
Stretchy (highly fertile)		
Dry		

Bleeding/Spotting

none ☐ light ☐ medium ☐ heavy ☐

symptoms
....

- ☐ Cramps/Aches & Pains
- ☐ Headaches/Brain fog
- ☐ Lack of concentration
- ☐ Breast tenderness
- ☐ Nausea
- ☐ Loss of appetite
- ☐ Fatigue
- ☐ Insomnia
- ☐ Other:

ovulation?
☐ Yes   ☐ No

OVARIAN PAIN/CYSTS(which side?):
_____

BASAL BODY TEMPERATURE:
_____

☐ Regular   ☐ Bloated   ☐ Constipated   ☐ Gassy

overall mood:

(happy)   (energetic)   (well-rested)   (calm)   (sad)

(irritable)   (depressed)   (anxious)   (wired)   (tired)

STRESS LEVEL/	low	medium	high
SEX or LIBIDO/	low	medium	high

SLEEP QUALITY	SUPPLEMENTS:

Nourishing Foods: _____

_____

Cravings: _____

_____

Exercise/Movement: _____

_____

_____

Workflow/Motivation: _____

_____

_____

month: ....

DAY/	CYCLE DAY/

CYCLE PHASE:

- ☐ Menstrual
- ☐ Follicular
- ☐ Ovulatory
- ☐ Luteal

MOON PHASE:

Cervical Mucus:
check 'yes' or 'no' in boxes below

	yes	no
Tacky		
Crumbly		
Rubbery		
Creamy		
White		
Slippery		
Stringy		
Stretchy (highly fertile)		
Dry		

Bleeding/Spotting

none ☐   light ☐   medium ☐   heavy ☐

symptoms
....

- ☐ Cramps/Aches & Pains
- ☐ Headaches/Brain fog
- ☐ Lack of concentration
- ☐ Breast tenderness
- ☐ Nausea
- ☐ Loss of appetite
- ☐ Fatigue
- ☐ Insomnia
- ☐ Other:

ovulation?
☐ Yes   ☐ No

OVARIAN PAIN/CYSTS(which side?):
_____

BASAL BODY TEMPERATURE:
_____

Digestion:

☐ Regular ☐ Bloated ☐ Constipated ☐ Gassy

overall mood:

(happy) (energetic) (well-rested) (calm) (sad)

(irritable) (depressed) (anxious) (wired) (tired)

STRESS LEVEL/	low	medium	high
SEX or LIBIDO/	low	medium	high

SLEEP QUALITY	SUPPLEMENTS:

Nourishing Foods: _____

Cravings: _____

Exercise/Movement: _____

Workflow/Motivation: _____

month: ....

DAY/	CYCLE DAY/

CYCLE PHASE:	MOON PHASE:
☐ Menstrual ☐ Follicular ☐ Ovulatory ☐ Luteal	

Cervical Mucus: ⬭ yes ⬭ no
check 'yes' or 'no' in boxes below

	yes	no
Tacky		
Crumbly		
Rubbery		
Creamy		
White		
Slippery		
Stringy		
Stretchy (highly fertile)		
Dry		

Bleeding/Spotting

none ☐   light ☐   medium ☐   heavy ☐

symptoms
....

☐ Cramps/Aches & Pains

☐ Headaches/Brain fog

☐ Lack of concentration

☐ Breast tenderness

☐ Nausea

☐ Loss of appetite

☐ Fatigue

☐ Insomnia

☐ Other:

ovulation?
☐ Yes   ☐ No

OVARIAN PAIN/CYSTS(which side?):

_____

BASAL BODY TEMPERATURE:

_____

☐ Regular ☐ Bloated ☐ Constipated ☐ Gassy

overall mood:

(happy) (energetic) (well-rested) (calm) (sad)

(irritable) (depressed) (anxious) (wired) (tired)

STRESS LEVEL/	low	medium	high
SEX or LIBIDO/	low	medium	high

SLEEP QUALITY	SUPPLEMENTS:

Nourishing Foods: _____

_____

Cravings: _____

_____

Exercise/Movement: _____

_____

_____

Workflow/Motivation: _____

_____

_____

weekly reflection:

....

SKIN FLUCTUATIONS:

☐ Normal

☐ Oily

☐ Dry

☐ Blemishes

☐ Dull

☐ Glowy

Trying to drink more water? Meal plan? Limit social media?

. . .

Record your weekly habits here.

↓

Happy Weekly Habits: _____

_____

_____

_____

_____

_____

_____

What worked well this week?	*What did not work well this week?*

me time moments.

Record any special self-care practices like meditation, gratitude journaling, epsom salt bath, manicure... whatever "me time" means to you.

Me Time Moments: _____

_____

_____

_____

_____

_____

_____

_____

YOU GOT THIS

My most memorable moment of the week was . . .

month: ....

DAY/	CYCLE DAY/

CYCLE PHASE:

☐ Menstrual
☐ Follicular
☐ Ovulatory
☐ Luteal

MOON PHASE:

Cervical Mucus: ⬭ yes ⬭ no
check 'yes' or 'no' in boxes below

	yes	no
Tacky		
Crumbly		
Rubbery		
Creamy		
White		
Slippery		
Stringy		
Stretchy (highly fertile)		
Dry		

Bleeding/Spotting

none ☐ light ☐ medium ☐ heavy ☐

symptoms
....

☐ Cramps/Aches & Pains
☐ Headaches/Brain fog
☐ Lack of concentration
☐ Breast tenderness
☐ Nausea
☐ Loss of appetite
☐ Fatigue
☐ Insomnia
☐ Other:

ovulation?
☐ Yes ☐ No

OVARIAN PAIN/CYSTS(which side?):
_____

BASAL BODY TEMPERATURE:
_____

Digestion:

☐ Regular ☐ Bloated ☐ Constipated ☐ Gassy

overall mood:

(happy) (energetic) (well-rested) (calm) (sad)

(irritable) (depressed) (anxious) (wired) (tired)

STRESS LEVEL/	low	medium	high
SEX or LIBIDO/	low	medium	high

SLEEP QUALITY	SUPPLEMENTS:

Nourishing Foods: _____

_____

Cravings: _____

_____

Exercise/Movement: _____

_____

_____

Workflow/Motivation: _____

_____

_____

month: ....

DAY/	CYCLE DAY/

CYCLE PHASE:

- ☐ Menstrual
- ☐ Follicular
- ☐ Ovulatory
- ☐ Luteal

MOON PHASE:

Cervical Mucus:
check 'yes' or 'no' in boxes below

	yes	no
Tacky		
Crumbly		
Rubbery		
Creamy		
White		
Slippery		
Stringy		
Stretchy (highly fertile)		
Dry		

Bleeding/Spotting
none ☐ light ☐ medium ☐ heavy ☐

symptoms
....

- ☐ Cramps/Aches & Pains
- ☐ Headaches/Brain fog
- ☐ Lack of concentration
- ☐ Breast tenderness
- ☐ Nausea
- ☐ Loss of appetite
- ☐ Fatigue
- ☐ Insomnia
- ☐ Other:

ovulation?
☐ Yes   ☐ No

OVARIAN PAIN/CYSTS(which side?):
_____

BASAL BODY TEMPERATURE:
_____

Digestion:

☐ Regular ☐ Bloated ☐ Constipated ☐ Gassy

overall mood:

happy	energetic	well-rested	calm	sad
irritable	depressed	anxious	wired	tired

STRESS LEVEL/	low	medium	high
SEX or LIBIDO/	low	medium	high

SLEEP QUALITY	**SUPPLEMENTS:**

Nourishing Foods: _____

_____

Cravings: _____

_____

Exercise/Movement: _____

_____

_____

Workflow/Motivation: _____

_____

_____

month:
....

DAY/	CYCLE DAY/

CYCLE PHASE:

- ☐ Menstrual
- ☐ Follicular
- ☐ Ovulatory
- ☐ Luteal

MOON PHASE:

Cervical Mucus:
check 'yes' or 'no' in boxes below

	yes	no
Tacky		
Crumbly		
Rubbery		
Creamy		
White		
Slippery		
Stringy		
Stretchy (highly fertile)		
Dry		

Bleeding/Spotting

none ☐   light ☐   medium ☐   heavy ☐

symptoms
....

- ☐ Cramps/Aches & Pains
- ☐ Headaches/Brain fog
- ☐ Lack of concentration
- ☐ Breast tenderness
- ☐ Nausea
- ☐ Loss of appetite
- ☐ Fatigue
- ☐ Insomnia
- ☐ Other:

ovulation?
☐ Yes   ☐ No

OVARIAN PAIN/CYSTS(which side?):
_____

BASAL BODY TEMPERATURE:
_____

☐ Regular   ☐ Bloated   ☐ Constipated   ☐ Gassy

overall mood:

happy	energetic	well-rested	calm	sad
irritable	depressed	anxious	wired	tired

STRESS LEVEL/	low	medium	high
SEX or LIBIDO/	low	medium	high

SLEEP QUALITY	SUPPLEMENTS:

Nourishing Foods: _____

Cravings: _____

Exercise/Movement: _____

Workflow/Motivation: _____

month: ....

DAY/	CYCLE DAY/

CYCLE PHASE:

- ☐ Menstrual
- ☐ Follicular
- ☐ Ovulatory
- ☐ Luteal

MOON PHASE:

Cervical Mucus: (yes) (no)
check 'yes' or 'no' in boxes below

	yes	no
Tacky		
Crumbly		
Rubbery		
Creamy		
White		
Slippery		
Stringy		
Stretchy (highly fertile)		
Dry		

Bleeding/Spotting

none ☐ light ☐ medium ☐ heavy ☐

symptoms
....

- ☐ Cramps/Aches & Pains
- ☐ Headaches/Brain fog
- ☐ Lack of concentration
- ☐ Breast tenderness
- ☐ Nausea
- ☐ Loss of appetite
- ☐ Fatigue
- ☐ Insomnia
- ☐ Other:

ovulation?
☐ Yes   ☐ No

OVARIAN PAIN/CYSTS(which side?):

BASAL BODY TEMPERATURE:

☐ Regular ☐ Bloated ☐ Constipated ☐ Gassy

overall mood:

happy	energetic	well-rested	calm	sad

irritable	depressed	anxious	wired	tired

STRESS LEVEL/	*low*	*medium*	*high*
SEX or LIBIDO/	*low*	*medium*	*high*

SLEEP QUALITY	**SUPPLEMENTS:**

Nourishing Foods: _____

_____

Cravings: _____

_____

Exercise/Movement: _____

_____

_____

Workflow/Motivation: _____

_____

_____

month: ....

DAY/	CYCLE DAY/

CYCLE PHASE:

- ☐ Menstrual
- ☐ Follicular
- ☐ Ovulatory
- ☐ Luteal

MOON PHASE:

Cervical Mucus: (yes)   (no)
check 'yes' or 'no' in boxes below

	yes	no
Tacky		
Crumbly		
Rubbery		
Creamy		
White		
Slippery		
Stringy		
Stretchy (highly fertile)		
Dry		

Bleeding/Spotting

none ☐   light ☐   medium ☐   heavy ☐

symptoms
....

- ☐ Cramps/Aches & Pains
- ☐ Headaches/Brain fog
- ☐ Lack of concentration
- ☐ Breast tenderness
- ☐ Nausea
- ☐ Loss of appetite
- ☐ Fatigue
- ☐ Insomnia
- ☐ Other:

ovulation?
☐ Yes   ☐ No

OVARIAN PAIN/CYSTS(which side?):

_____

BASAL BODY TEMPERATURE:

_____

☐ Regular ☐ Bloated ☐ Constipated ☐ Gassy

overall mood:

(happy) (energetic) (well-rested) (calm) (sad)

(irritable) (depressed) (anxious) (wired) (tired)

STRESS LEVEL/	low	medium	high
SEX or LIBIDO/	low	medium	high

SLEEP QUALITY	SUPPLEMENTS:

Nourishing Foods: _____

_____

Cravings: _____

_____

Exercise/Movement: _____

_____

_____

Workflow/Motivation: _____

_____

_____

month: ....

DAY/	CYCLE DAY/

CYCLE PHASE:

- ☐ Menstrual
- ☐ Follicular
- ☐ Ovulatory
- ☐ Luteal

MOON PHASE:

Cervical Mucus: ⬭ yes ⬭ no
check 'yes' or 'no' in boxes below

Tacky		
Crumbly		
Rubbery		
Creamy		
White		
Slippery		
Stringy		
Stretchy (highly fertile)		
Dry		

Bleeding/Spotting

none ☐   light ☐   medium ☐   heavy ☐

symptoms
....

- ☐ Cramps/Aches & Pains
- ☐ Headaches/Brain fog
- ☐ Lack of concentration
- ☐ Breast tenderness
- ☐ Nausea
- ☐ Loss of appetite
- ☐ Fatigue
- ☐ Insomnia
- ☐ Other:

ovulation?
☐ Yes   ☐ No

OVARIAN PAIN/CYSTS(which side?):

_____

BASAL BODY TEMPERATURE:

_____

☐ Regular ☐ Bloated ☐ Constipated ☐ Gassy

overall mood:

happy	energetic	well-rested	calm	sad
irritable	depressed	anxious	wired	tired

STRESS LEVEL/	low	medium	high
SEX or LIBIDO/	low	medium	high

SLEEP QUALITY	**SUPPLEMENTS:**

Nourishing Foods: _____

Cravings: _____

Exercise/Movement: _____

Workflow/Motivation: _____

month: ....

DAY/	CYCLE DAY/

CYCLE PHASE:

- ☐ Menstrual
- ☐ Follicular
- ☐ Ovulatory
- ☐ Luteal

MOON PHASE:

Cervical Mucus:
check 'yes' or 'no' in boxes below

(yes) (no)

	yes	no
Tacky		
Crumbly		
Rubbery		
Creamy		
White		
Slippery		
Stringy		
Stretchy (highly fertile)		
Dry		

Bleeding/Spotting

none ☐   light ☐   medium ☐   heavy ☐

symptoms
....

- ☐ Cramps/Aches & Pains
- ☐ Headaches/Brain fog
- ☐ Lack of concentration
- ☐ Breast tenderness
- ☐ Nausea
- ☐ Loss of appetite
- ☐ Fatigue
- ☐ Insomnia
- ☐ Other:

ovulation?

☐ Yes   ☐ No

OVARIAN PAIN/CYSTS(which side?):

_____

BASAL BODY TEMPERATURE:

_____

Digestion:

☐ Regular ☐ Bloated ☐ Constipated ☐ Gassy

overall mood:

| happy | energetic | well-rested | calm | sad |

| irritable | depressed | anxious | wired | tired |

STRESS LEVEL/	low	medium	high
SEX or LIBIDO/	low	medium	high

SLEEP QUALITY	**SUPPLEMENTS:**

Nourishing Foods: _____

_____

Cravings: _____

_____

Exercise/Movement: _____

_____

_____

Workflow/Motivation: _____

_____

_____

weekly reflection:

SKIN FLUCTUATIONS:

- ☐ Normal
- ☐ Oily
- ☐ Dry
- ☐ Blemishes
- ☐ Dull
- ☐ Glowy

Trying to drink more water? Meal plan? Limit social media?

. . .

Record your weekly habits here.

↓

Happy Weekly Habits: _____

_____

_____

_____

_____

_____

_____

What worked well this week?	*What did not work well this week?*

me time moments.

Record any special self-care practices like meditation,
gratitude journaling, epsom salt bath, manicure...
whatever "me time" means to you.

Me Time Moments: _____

_____

_____

_____

_____

_____

_____

YOU
GOT
THIS

My most memorable moment
of the week was . . .

_____

_____

_____

_____

_____

_____

_____

_____

month: ....

DAY/	CYCLE DAY/

CYCLE PHASE:	MOON PHASE:
☐ Menstrual ☐ Follicular ☐ Ovulatory ☐ Luteal	

Cervical Mucus: (yes) (no)
check 'yes' or 'no' in boxes below

	yes	no
Tacky		
Crumbly		
Rubbery		
Creamy		
White		
Slippery		
Stringy		
Stretchy (highly fertile)		
Dry		

Bleeding/Spotting

none ☐ light ☐ medium ☐ heavy ☐

symptoms

....

☐ Cramps/Aches & Pains

☐ Headaches/Brain fog

☐ Lack of concentration

☐ Breast tenderness

☐ Nausea

☐ Loss of appetite

☐ Fatigue

☐ Insomnia

☐ Other:

ovulation?

☐ Yes ☐ No

OVARIAN PAIN/CYSTS(which side?):
_____

BASAL BODY TEMPERATURE:
_____

☐ Regular   ☐ Bloated   ☐ Constipated   ☐ Gassy

overall mood:

(happy)   (energetic)   (well-rested)   (calm)   (sad)

(irritable)   (depressed)   (anxious)   (wired)   (tired)

STRESS LEVEL/	low	medium	high
SEX or LIBIDO/	low	medium	high

SLEEP QUALITY	**SUPPLEMENTS:**

Nourishing Foods: _____

_____

Cravings: _____

_____

Exercise/Movement: _____

_____

_____

Workflow/Motivation: _____

_____

_____

month: ....

DAY/	CYCLE DAY/

CYCLE PHASE:

- ❑ Menstrual
- ❑ Follicular
- ❑ Ovulatory
- ❑ Luteal

MOON PHASE:

Cervical Mucus:
check 'yes' or 'no' in boxes below

	yes	no
Tacky		
Crumbly		
Rubbery		
Creamy		
White		
Slippery		
Stringy		
Stretchy (highly fertile)		
Dry		

Bleeding/Spotting

none ❑ light ❑ medium ❑ heavy ❑

symptoms
....

- ❑ Cramps/Aches & Pains
- ❑ Headaches/Brain fog
- ❑ Lack of concentration
- ❑ Breast tenderness
- ❑ Nausea
- ❑ Loss of appetite
- ❑ Fatigue
- ❑ Insomnia
- ❑ Other:

ovulation?
❑ Yes   ❑ No

OVARIAN PAIN/CYSTS(which side?):

_____

BASAL BODY TEMPERATURE:

_____

☐ Regular ☐ Bloated ☐ Constipated ☐ Gassy

overall mood:

(happy) (energetic) (well-rested) (calm) (sad)

(irritable) (depressed) (anxious) (wired) (tired)

STRESS LEVEL/	*low*	*medium*	*high*
SEX or LIBIDO/	*low*	*medium*	*high*

SLEEP QUALITY	**SUPPLEMENTS:**

Nourishing Foods: _____

_____

Cravings: _____

_____

Exercise/Movement: _____

_____

_____

Workflow/Motivation: _____

_____

_____

month:

DAY/	CYCLE DAY/

CYCLE PHASE:

☐ Menstrual
☐ Follicular
☐ Ovulatory
☐ Luteal

MOON PHASE:

Cervical Mucus:
check 'yes' or 'no' in boxes below

(yes) (no)

	yes	no
Tacky		
Crumbly		
Rubbery		
Creamy		
White		
Slippery		
Stringy		
Stretchy (highly fertile)		
Dry		

Bleeding/Spotting

none ☐ light ☐ medium ☐ heavy ☐

symptoms

☐ Cramps/Aches & Pains
☐ Headaches/Brain fog
☐ Lack of concentration
☐ Breast tenderness
☐ Nausea
☐ Loss of appetite
☐ Fatigue
☐ Insomnia
☐ Other:

ovulation?
☐ Yes   ☐ No

OVARIAN PAIN/CYSTS(which side?):

BASAL BODY TEMPERATURE:

Digestion:

☐ Regular ☐ Bloated ☐ Constipated ☐ Gassy

overall mood:

| happy | energetic | well-rested | calm | sad |

| irritable | depressed | anxious | wired | tired |

| **STRESS LEVEL/** | low | medium | high |
| **SEX or LIBIDO/** | low | medium | high |

SLEEP QUALITY

SUPPLEMENTS:

Nourishing Foods: _____

_____

Cravings: _____

_____

Exercise/Movement: _____

_____

_____

Workflow/Motivation: _____

_____

_____

month: ....

DAY/	CYCLE DAY/

CYCLE PHASE:

- ☐ Menstrual
- ☐ Follicular
- ☐ Ovulatory
- ☐ Luteal

MOON PHASE:

Cervical Mucus:
check 'yes' or 'no' in boxes below

	yes	no
Tacky		
Crumbly		
Rubbery		
Creamy		
White		
Slippery		
Stringy		
Stretchy (highly fertile)		
Dry		

Bleeding/Spotting

none ☐ light ☐ medium ☐ heavy ☐

symptoms
....

- ☐ Cramps/Aches & Pains
- ☐ Headaches/Brain fog
- ☐ Lack of concentration
- ☐ Breast tenderness
- ☐ Nausea
- ☐ Loss of appetite
- ☐ Fatigue
- ☐ Insomnia
- ☐ Other:

ovulation?
☐ Yes   ☐ No

OVARIAN PAIN/CYSTS(which side?):
_____

BASAL BODY TEMPERATURE:
_____

Digestion:

☐ Regular   ☐ Bloated   ☐ Constipated   ☐ Gassy

overall mood:

(happy) (energetic) (well-rested) (calm) (sad)

(irritable) (depressed) (anxious) (wired) (tired)

STRESS LEVEL/	low	medium	high
SEX or LIBIDO/	low	medium	high

SLEEP QUALITY	SUPPLEMENTS:

Nourishing Foods: _____

_____

Cravings: _____

_____

Exercise/Movement: _____

_____

_____

Workflow/Motivation: _____

_____

_____

month: ....

DAY/	CYCLE DAY/

CYCLE PHASE:

- ☐ Menstrual
- ☐ Follicular
- ☐ Ovulatory
- ☐ Luteal

MOON PHASE:

Cervical Mucus:
check 'yes' or 'no' in boxes below   (yes) (no)

	yes	no
Tacky		
Crumbly		
Rubbery		
Creamy		
White		
Slippery		
Stringy		
Stretchy (highly fertile)		
Dry		

Bleeding/Spotting

none ☐   light ☐   medium ☐   heavy ☐

symptoms
....

- ☐ Cramps/Aches & Pains
- ☐ Headaches/Brain fog
- ☐ Lack of concentration
- ☐ Breast tenderness
- ☐ Nausea
- ☐ Loss of appetite
- ☐ Fatigue
- ☐ Insomnia
- ☐ Other:

ovulation?
☐ Yes   ☐ No

OVARIAN PAIN/CYSTS(which side?):
_____

BASAL BODY TEMPERATURE:
_____

Digestion:

☐ Regular ☐ Bloated ☐ Constipated ☐ Gassy

overall mood:

(happy) (energetic) (well-rested) (calm) (sad)

(irritable) (depressed) (anxious) (wired) (tired)

STRESS LEVEL/	low	medium	high
SEX or LIBIDO/	low	medium	high

SLEEP QUALITY	**SUPPLEMENTS:**

Nourishing Foods: _____

Cravings: _____

Exercise/Movement: _____

Workflow/Motivation: _____

month: ....

DAY/	CYCLE DAY/

CYCLE PHASE:

☐ Menstrual
☐ Follicular
☐ Ovulatory
☐ Luteal

MOON PHASE:

Cervical Mucus:
check 'yes' or 'no' in boxes below   (yes)   (no)

Tacky		
Crumbly		
Rubbery		
Creamy		
White		
Slippery		
Stringy		
Stretchy (highly fertile)		
Dry		

Bleeding/Spotting

none ☐   light ☐   medium ☐   heavy ☐

symptoms
....

☐ Cramps/Aches & Pains
☐ Headaches/Brain fog
☐ Lack of concentration
☐ Breast tenderness
☐ Nausea
☐ Loss of appetite
☐ Fatigue
☐ Insomnia
☐ Other:

ovulation?
☐ Yes   ☐ No

OVARIAN PAIN/CYSTS(which side?):
_____

BASAL BODY TEMPERATURE:

Digestion:

☐ Regular ☐ Bloated ☐ Constipated ☐ Gassy

overall mood:

(happy) (energetic) (well-rested) (calm) (sad)

(irritable) (depressed) (anxious) (wired) (tired)

STRESS LEVEL/	low	medium	high
SEX or LIBIDO/	low	medium	high

SLEEP QUALITY	SUPPLEMENTS:

Nourishing Foods: _____

Cravings: _____

Exercise/Movement: _____

Workflow/Motivation: _____

month: ....

DAY/	CYCLE DAY/

CYCLE PHASE:

- ❑ Menstrual
- ❑ Follicular
- ❑ Ovulatory
- ❑ Luteal

MOON PHASE:

Cervical Mucus: (yes) (no)
check 'yes' or 'no' in boxes below

	yes	no
Tacky		
Crumbly		
Rubbery		
Creamy		
White		
Slippery		
Stringy		
Stretchy (highly fertile)		
Dry		

Bleeding/Spotting

none ❑   light ❑   medium ❑   heavy ❑

symptoms
....

- ❑ Cramps/Aches & Pains
- ❑ Headaches/Brain fog
- ❑ Lack of concentration
- ❑ Breast tenderness
- ❑ Nausea
- ❑ Loss of appetite
- ❑ Fatigue
- ❑ Insomnia
- ❑ Other:

ovulation?
❑ Yes   ❑ No

OVARIAN PAIN/CYSTS(which side?):

_____

BASAL BODY TEMPERATURE:

_____

Digestion:

☐ Regular ☐ Bloated ☐ Constipated ☐ Gassy

overall mood:

happy   energetic   well-rested   calm   sad

irritable   depressed   anxious   wired   tired

STRESS LEVEL/	low	medium	high
SEX or LIBIDO/	low	medium	high

SLEEP QUALITY	SUPPLEMENTS:

Nourishing Foods: _____

Cravings: _____

Exercise/Movement: _____

Workflow/Motivation: _____

weekly reflection:

SKIN FLUCTUATIONS:

- ☐ Normal
- ☐ Oily
- ☐ Dry
- ☐ Blemishes
- ☐ Dull
- ☐ Glowy

Trying to drink more water? Meal plan? Limit social media?

. . .

Record your weekly habits here.

↓

Happy Weekly Habits: _____

_____

_____

_____

_____

_____

_____

What worked well this week?	*What did not work well this week?*

me time moments.

Record any special self-care practices like meditation,
gratitude journaling, epsom salt bath, manicure...
whatever "me time" means to you.

Me Time Moments: _____

_____

_____

_____

_____

_____

_____

_____

YOU
GOT
THIS

My most memorable moment of the week was . . .

_____

_____

_____

_____

_____

_____

_____

_____

month: ....

DAY/	CYCLE DAY/

CYCLE PHASE:

- ☐ Menstrual
- ☐ Follicular
- ☐ Ovulatory
- ☐ Luteal

MOON PHASE:

Cervical Mucus:
check 'yes' or 'no' in boxes below

	yes	no
Tacky		
Crumbly		
Rubbery		
Creamy		
White		
Slippery		
Stringy		
Stretchy (highly fertile)		
Dry		

Bleeding/Spotting

none ☐ light ☐ medium ☐ heavy ☐

symptoms
....

- ☐ Cramps/Aches & Pains
- ☐ Headaches/Brain fog
- ☐ Lack of concentration
- ☐ Breast tenderness
- ☐ Nausea
- ☐ Loss of appetite
- ☐ Fatigue
- ☐ Insomnia
- ☐ Other:

ovulation?

☐ Yes   ☐ No

OVARIAN PAIN/CYSTS(which side?):

_____

BASAL BODY TEMPERATURE:

_____

☐ Regular ☐ Bloated ☐ Constipated ☐ Gassy

overall mood:

(happy) (energetic) (well-rested) (calm) (sad)

(irritable) (depressed) (anxious) (wired) (tired)

STRESS LEVEL/	low	medium	high
SEX or LIBIDO/	low	medium	high

SLEEP QUALITY	SUPPLEMENTS:

Nourishing Foods: _____

_____

Cravings: _____

_____

Exercise/Movement: _____

_____

Workflow/Motivation: _____

_____

_____

month: ....

DAY/	CYCLE DAY/

CYCLE PHASE:

- ☐ Menstrual
- ☐ Follicular
- ☐ Ovulatory
- ☐ Luteal

MOON PHASE:

Cervical Mucus:
check 'yes' or 'no' in boxes below

	yes	no
Tacky		
Crumbly		
Rubbery		
Creamy		
White		
Slippery		
Stringy		
Stretchy (highly fertile)		
Dry		

Bleeding/Spotting

none ☐   light ☐   medium ☐   heavy ☐

symptoms
....

- ☐ Cramps/Aches & Pains
- ☐ Headaches/Brain fog
- ☐ Lack of concentration
- ☐ Breast tenderness
- ☐ Nausea
- ☐ Loss of appetite
- ☐ Fatigue
- ☐ Insomnia
- ☐ Other:

ovulation?

☐ Yes   ☐ No

OVARIAN PAIN/CYSTS(which side?):
_____

BASAL BODY TEMPERATURE:
_____

Digestion:

☐ Regular ☐ Bloated ☐ Constipated ☐ Gassy

overall mood:

(happy) (energetic) (well-rested) (calm) (sad)

(irritable) (depressed) (anxious) (wired) (tired)

STRESS LEVEL/	low	medium	high
SEX or LIBIDO/	low	medium	high

SLEEP QUALITY	SUPPLEMENTS:

Nourishing Foods: _____

_____

Cravings: _____

_____

Exercise/Movement: _____

_____

_____

Workflow/Motivation: _____

_____

_____

month: ....

DAY/	CYCLE DAY/

CYCLE PHASE:	**MOON PHASE:**
☐ Menstrual ☐ Follicular ☐ Ovulatory ☐ Luteal	

Cervical Mucus: ⬭yes ⬭no
check 'yes' or 'no' in boxes below

	yes	no
Tacky		
Crumbly		
Rubbery		
Creamy		
White		
Slippery		
Stringy		
Stretchy (highly fertile)		
Dry		

Bleeding/Spotting

none ☐ light ☐ medium ☐ heavy ☐

symptoms
....

☐ Cramps/Aches & Pains

☐ Headaches/Brain fog

☐ Lack of concentration

☐ Breast tenderness

☐ Nausea

☐ Loss of appetite

☐ Fatigue

☐ Insomnia

☐ Other:

ovulation?
☐ Yes   ☐ No

OVARIAN PAIN/CYSTS(which side?):

_____

BASAL BODY TEMPERATURE:

_____

Digestion:

☐ Regular ☐ Bloated ☐ Constipated ☐ Gassy

overall mood:

happy	energetic	well-rested	calm	sad
irritable	depressed	anxious	wired	tired

STRESS LEVEL/	low	medium	high
SEX or LIBIDO/	low	medium	high

SLEEP QUALITY	**SUPPLEMENTS:**

Nourishing Foods: _____

_____

Cravings: _____

_____

Exercise/Movement: _____

_____

_____

Workflow/Motivation: _____

_____

_____

month: ....

DAY/	CYCLE DAY/

CYCLE PHASE:

- ☐ Menstrual
- ☐ Follicular
- ☐ Ovulatory
- ☐ Luteal

MOON PHASE:

Cervical Mucus: ⬭ yes ⬭ no
check 'yes' or 'no' in boxes below

	yes	no
Tacky		
Crumbly		
Rubbery		
Creamy		
White		
Slippery		
Stringy		
Stretchy (highly fertile)		
Dry		

Bleeding/Spotting

none ☐ light ☐ medium ☐ heavy ☐

symptoms
....

- ☐ Cramps/Aches & Pains
- ☐ Headaches/Brain fog
- ☐ Lack of concentration
- ☐ Breast tenderness
- ☐ Nausea
- ☐ Loss of appetite
- ☐ Fatigue
- ☐ Insomnia
- ☐ Other:

ovulation?
☐ Yes   ☐ No

OVARIAN PAIN/CYSTS(which side?):
_____

BASAL BODY TEMPERATURE:
_____

☐ Regular　☐ Bloated　☐ Constipated　☐ Gassy

overall mood:

| (happy) | (energetic) | (well-rested) | (calm) | (sad) |

| (irritable) | (depressed) | (anxious) | (wired) | (tired) |

| **STRESS LEVEL/** | low | medium | high |
| **SEX or LIBIDO/** | low | medium | high |

SLEEP QUALITY	**SUPPLEMENTS:**

Nourishing Foods: _____

Cravings: _____

Exercise/Movement: _____

Workflow/Motivation: _____

month: ....

DAY/	CYCLE DAY/

CYCLE PHASE:	MOON PHASE:
❑ Menstrual ❑ Follicular ❑ Ovulatory ❑ Luteal	

Cervical Mucus:
check 'yes' or 'no' in boxes below   ⬭ yes   ⬭ no

Tacky		
Crumbly		
Rubbery		
Creamy		
White		
Slippery		
Stringy		
Stretchy (highly fertile)		
Dry		

Bleeding/Spotting

none ❑   light ❑   medium ❑   heavy ❑

symptoms
....

❑ Cramps/Aches & Pains

❑ Headaches/Brain fog

❑ Lack of concentration

❑ Breast tenderness

❑ Nausea

❑ Loss of appetite

❑ Fatigue

❑ Insomnia

❑ Other:

ovulation?
❑ Yes   ❑ No

OVARIAN PAIN/CYSTS(which side?):
_____

BASAL BODY TEMPERATURE:
_____

☐ Regular   ☐ Bloated   ☐ Constipated   ☐ Gassy

overall mood:

(happy)   (energetic)   (well-rested)   (calm)   (sad)

(irritable)   (depressed)   (anxious)   (wired)   (tired)

STRESS LEVEL/	low	medium	high
SEX or LIBIDO/	low	medium	high

SLEEP QUALITY	SUPPLEMENTS:

Nourishing Foods: _____

_____

Cravings: _____

_____

Exercise/Movement: _____

_____

_____

Workflow/Motivation: _____

_____

_____

month: ....

DAY/	CYCLE DAY/

CYCLE PHASE:

- ☐ Menstrual
- ☐ Follicular
- ☐ Ovulatory
- ☐ Luteal

MOON PHASE:

Cervical Mucus: (yes) (no)
check 'yes' or 'no' in boxes below

	yes	no
Tacky		
Crumbly		
Rubbery		
Creamy		
White		
Slippery		
Stringy		
Stretchy (highly fertile)		
Dry		

Bleeding/Spotting

none ☐   light ☐   medium ☐   heavy ☐

symptoms
....

- ☐ Cramps/Aches & Pains
- ☐ Headaches/Brain fog
- ☐ Lack of concentration
- ☐ Breast tenderness
- ☐ Nausea
- ☐ Loss of appetite
- ☐ Fatigue
- ☐ Insomnia
- ☐ Other:

ovulation?
☐ Yes   ☐ No

OVARIAN PAIN/CYSTS(which side?):
_____

BASAL BODY TEMPERATURE:
_____

Digestion:

☐ Regular ☐ Bloated ☐ Constipated ☐ Gassy

overall mood:

(happy) (energetic) (well-rested) (calm) (sad)

(irritable) (depressed) (anxious) (wired) (tired)

STRESS LEVEL/	low	medium	high
SEX or LIBIDO/	low	medium	high

SLEEP QUALITY	SUPPLEMENTS:

Nourishing Foods: _____

_____

Cravings: _____

_____

Exercise/Movement: _____

_____

_____

Workflow/Motivation: _____

_____

_____

month:

DAY/	CYCLE DAY/

CYCLE PHASE:

- ☐ Menstrual
- ☐ Follicular
- ☐ Ovulatory
- ☐ Luteal

MOON PHASE:

Cervical Mucus:
check 'yes' or 'no' in boxes below   ⬭ yes   ⬭ no

Tacky		
Crumbly		
Rubbery		
Creamy		
White		
Slippery		
Stringy		
Stretchy (highly fertile)		
Dry		

Bleeding/Spotting

none ☐   light ☐   medium ☐   heavy ☐

symptoms

- ☐ Cramps/Aches & Pains
- ☐ Headaches/Brain fog
- ☐ Lack of concentration
- ☐ Breast tenderness
- ☐ Nausea
- ☐ Loss of appetite
- ☐ Fatigue
- ☐ Insomnia
- ☐ Other:

ovulation?
☐ Yes   ☐ No

OVARIAN PAIN/CYSTS(which side?):

BASAL BODY TEMPERATURE:

Digestion:

☐ Regular ☐ Bloated ☐ Constipated ☐ Gassy

overall mood:

(happy) (energetic) (well-rested) (calm) (sad)

(irritable) (depressed) (anxious) (wired) (tired)

STRESS LEVEL/	low	medium	high
SEX or LIBIDO/	low	medium	high

SLEEP QUALITY	SUPPLEMENTS:

Nourishing Foods: _____

_____

Cravings: _____

_____

Exercise/Movement: _____

_____

_____

Workflow/Motivation: _____

_____

_____

weekly reflection:

SKIN FLUCTUATIONS:

- [ ] Normal
- [ ] Oily
- [ ] Dry
- [ ] Blemishes
- [ ] Dull
- [ ] Glowy

Trying to drink more water? Meal plan? Limit social media?

. . .

Record your weekly habits here.

↓

Happy Weekly Habits: _____

_____

_____

_____

_____

_____

What worked well this week?	*What did not work well this week?*

me time moments.

Record any special self-care practices like meditation, gratitude journaling, epsom salt bath, manicure... whatever "me time" means to you.

Me Time Moments: _____

_____

_____

_____

_____

_____

_____

_____

_____

YOU
GOT
THIS

My most memorable moment of the week was . . .

_____

_____

_____

_____

_____

_____

_____

_____

month: ....

DAY/	CYCLE DAY/

CYCLE PHASE:

- ☐ Menstrual
- ☐ Follicular
- ☐ Ovulatory
- ☐ Luteal

MOON PHASE:

Cervical Mucus: ⟨yes⟩ ⟨no⟩
check 'yes' or 'no' in boxes below

	yes	no
Tacky		
Crumbly		
Rubbery		
Creamy		
White		
Slippery		
Stringy		
Stretchy (highly fertile)		
Dry		

Bleeding/Spotting

none ☐ light ☐ medium ☐ heavy ☐

symptoms
....

- ☐ Cramps/Aches & Pains
- ☐ Headaches/Brain fog
- ☐ Lack of concentration
- ☐ Breast tenderness
- ☐ Nausea
- ☐ Loss of appetite
- ☐ Fatigue
- ☐ Insomnia
- ☐ Other:

ovulation?
☐ Yes   ☐ No

OVARIAN PAIN/CYSTS(which side?):

_____

BASAL BODY TEMPERATURE:

_____

Digestion:

☐ Regular ☐ Bloated ☐ Constipated ☐ Gassy

overall mood:

| happy | energetic | well-rested | calm | sad |

| irritable | depressed | anxious | wired | tired |

| **STRESS LEVEL/** | low | medium | high |
| **SEX or LIBIDO/** | low | medium | high |

SLEEP QUALITY	**SUPPLEMENTS:**

Nourishing Foods: _____

Cravings: _____

Exercise/Movement: _____

Workflow/Motivation: _____

month: ....

DAY/	CYCLE DAY/

CYCLE PHASE:

- ☐ Menstrual
- ☐ Follicular
- ☐ Ovulatory
- ☐ Luteal

MOON PHASE:

Cervical Mucus:
check 'yes' or 'no' in boxes below   (yes)   (no)

	yes	no
Tacky		
Crumbly		
Rubbery		
Creamy		
White		
Slippery		
Stringy		
Stretchy (highly fertile)		
Dry		

Bleeding/Spotting

none ☐   light ☐   medium ☐   heavy ☐

symptoms
....

- ☐ Cramps/Aches & Pains
- ☐ Headaches/Brain fog
- ☐ Lack of concentration
- ☐ Breast tenderness
- ☐ Nausea
- ☐ Loss of appetite
- ☐ Fatigue
- ☐ Insomnia
- ☐ Other:

ovulation?
☐ Yes   ☐ No

OVARIAN PAIN/CYSTS(which side?):

_____

BASAL BODY TEMPERATURE:

_____

Digestion:

☐ Regular ☐ Bloated ☐ Constipated ☐ Gassy

overall mood:

(happy) (energetic) (well-rested) (calm) (sad)

(irritable) (depressed) (anxious) (wired) (tired)

| STRESS LEVEL/ | low | medium | high |
| SEX or LIBIDO/ | low | medium | high |

SLEEP QUALITY

SUPPLEMENTS:

Nourishing Foods: _____

Cravings: _____

Exercise/Movement: _____

Workflow/Motivation: _____

month: ....

DAY/	CYCLE DAY/

CYCLE PHASE:	MOON PHASE:
☐ Menstrual ☐ Follicular ☐ Ovulatory ☐ Luteal	

Cervical Mucus: ⟨ yes ⟩ ⟨ no ⟩
check 'yes' or 'no' in boxes below

	yes	no
Tacky		
Crumbly		
Rubbery		
Creamy		
White		
Slippery		
Stringy		
Stretchy (highly fertile)		
Dry		

Bleeding/Spotting
none ☐   light ☐   medium ☐   heavy ☐

symptoms
....

☐ Cramps/Aches & Pains

☐ Headaches/Brain fog

☐ Lack of concentration

☐ Breast tenderness

☐ Nausea

☐ Loss of appetite

☐ Fatigue

☐ Insomnia

☐ Other:

ovulation?
☐ Yes   ☐ No

OVARIAN PAIN/CYSTS(which side?):
_____

BASAL BODY TEMPERATURE:
_____

☐ Regular   ☐ Bloated   ☐ Constipated   ☐ Gassy

overall mood:

(happy)   (energetic)   (well-rested)   (calm)   (sad)

(irritable)   (depressed)   (anxious)   (wired)   (tired)

STRESS LEVEL/	low	medium	high
SEX or LIBIDO/	low	medium	high

SLEEP QUALITY	SUPPLEMENTS:

Nourishing Foods: _____

_____

Cravings: _____

_____

Exercise/Movement: _____

_____

_____

Workflow/Motivation: _____

_____

_____

month: ....

DAY/	CYCLE DAY/

CYCLE PHASE:	MOON PHASE:
☐ Menstrual ☐ Follicular ☐ Ovulatory ☐ Luteal	

Cervical Mucus:
check 'yes' or 'no' in boxes below   ⬭ yes   ⬭ no

	yes	no
Tacky		
Crumbly		
Rubbery		
Creamy		
White		
Slippery		
Stringy		
Stretchy (highly fertile)		
Dry		

Bleeding/Spotting
none ☐   light ☐   medium ☐   heavy ☐

symptoms
....

☐ Cramps/Aches & Pains

☐ Headaches/Brain fog

☐ Lack of concentration

☐ Breast tenderness

☐ Nausea

☐ Loss of appetite

☐ Fatigue

☐ Insomnia

☐ Other:

ovulation?
☐ Yes   ☐ No

OVARIAN PAIN/CYSTS(which side?):

BASAL BODY TEMPERATURE:

Digestion:

☐ Regular ☐ Bloated ☐ Constipated ☐ Gassy

overall mood:

| happy | energetic | well-rested | calm | sad |

| irritable | depressed | anxious | wired | tired |

| **STRESS LEVEL/** | low | medium | high |
| **SEX or LIBIDO/** | low | medium | high |

| **SLEEP QUALITY** | **SUPPLEMENTS:** |

Nourishing Foods: _____

Cravings: _____

Exercise/Movement: _____

Workflow/Motivation: _____

month: ....

DAY/	CYCLE DAY/

CYCLE PHASE:

- ☐ Menstrual
- ☐ Follicular
- ☐ Ovulatory
- ☐ Luteal

MOON PHASE:

Cervical Mucus: ⟨ yes ⟩ ⟨ no ⟩
check 'yes' or 'no' in boxes below

	yes	no
Tacky		
Crumbly		
Rubbery		
Creamy		
White		
Slippery		
Stringy		
Stretchy (highly fertile)		
Dry		

Bleeding/Spotting

none ☐ light ☐ medium ☐ heavy ☐

symptoms

....

- ☐ Cramps/Aches & Pains
- ☐ Headaches/Brain fog
- ☐ Lack of concentration
- ☐ Breast tenderness
- ☐ Nausea
- ☐ Loss of appetite
- ☐ Fatigue
- ☐ Insomnia
- ☐ Other:

ovulation?

☐ Yes   ☐ No

OVARIAN PAIN/CYSTS(which side?):
_____

BASAL BODY TEMPERATURE:
_____

Digestion:

☐ Regular ☐ Bloated ☐ Constipated ☐ Gassy

overall mood:

(happy) (energetic) (well-rested) (calm) (sad)

(irritable) (depressed) (anxious) (wired) (tired)

STRESS LEVEL/	low	medium	high
SEX or LIBIDO/	low	medium	high

SLEEP QUALITY	SUPPLEMENTS:

Nourishing Foods: _____

Cravings: _____

Exercise/Movement: _____

Workflow/Motivation: _____

month: ....

DAY/	CYCLE DAY/

CYCLE PHASE:

- ☐ Menstrual
- ☐ Follicular
- ☐ Ovulatory
- ☐ Luteal

MOON PHASE:

Cervical Mucus:
check 'yes' or 'no' in boxes below

	yes	no
Tacky		
Crumbly		
Rubbery		
Creamy		
White		
Slippery		
Stringy		
Stretchy (highly fertile)		
Dry		

Bleeding/Spotting

none ☐ light ☐ medium ☐ heavy ☐

symptoms
....

- ☐ Cramps/Aches & Pains
- ☐ Headaches/Brain fog
- ☐ Lack of concentration
- ☐ Breast tenderness
- ☐ Nausea
- ☐ Loss of appetite
- ☐ Fatigue
- ☐ Insomnia
- ☐ Other:

ovulation?
☐ Yes   ☐ No

OVARIAN PAIN/CYSTS(which side?):
_____

BASAL BODY TEMPERATURE:
_____

☐ Regular ☐ Bloated ☐ Constipated ☐ Gassy

overall mood:

(happy) (energetic) (well-rested) (calm) (sad)

(irritable) (depressed) (anxious) (wired) (tired)

STRESS LEVEL/	low	medium	high
SEX or LIBIDO/	low	medium	high

SLEEP QUALITY	SUPPLEMENTS:

Nourishing Foods: _____

_____

Cravings: _____

_____

Exercise/Movement: _____

_____

_____

Workflow/Motivation: _____

_____

_____

month: ....

DAY/	CYCLE DAY/

CYCLE PHASE:	**MOON PHASE:**
☐ Menstrual ☐ Follicular ☐ Ovulatory ☐ Luteal	

Cervical Mucus: (yes)   (no)

check 'yes' or 'no' in boxes below

	yes	no
Tacky		
Crumbly		
Rubbery		
Creamy		
White		
Slippery		
Stringy		
Stretchy (highly fertile)		
Dry		

Bleeding/Spotting

none ☐   light ☐   medium ☐   heavy ☐

symptoms
....

☐   Cramps/Aches & Pains

☐   Headaches/Brain fog

☐   Lack of concentration

☐   Breast tenderness

☐   Nausea

☐   Loss of appetite

☐   Fatigue

☐   Insomnia

☐   Other:

ovulation?
☐ Yes   ☐ No

OVARIAN PAIN/CYSTS(which side?):

_____

BASAL BODY TEMPERATURE:

_____

Digestion:

☐ Regular   ☐ Bloated   ☐ Constipated   ☐ Gassy

overall mood:

(happy)   (energetic)   (well-rested)   (calm)   (sad)

(irritable)   (depressed)   (anxious)   (wired)   (tired)

STRESS LEVEL/	low	medium	high
SEX or LIBIDO/	low	medium	high

SLEEP QUALITY	SUPPLEMENTS:

Nourishing Foods: _____

_____

Cravings: _____

_____

Exercise/Movement: _____

_____

_____

Workflow/Motivation: _____

_____

_____

weekly reflection:

SKIN FLUCTUATIONS:

☐ Normal

☐ Oily

☐ Dry

☐ Blemishes

☐ Dull

☐ Glowy

Trying to drink more water? Meal plan? Limit social media?

. . .

Record your weekly habits here.

↓

Happy Weekly Habits: _____

_____

_____

_____

_____

_____

_____

What worked well this week?

What did not work well this week?

me time moments.

Record any special self-care practices like meditation, gratitude journaling, epsom salt bath, manicure... whatever "me time" means to you.

Me Time Moments: _____

_____

_____

_____

_____

_____

_____

_____

_____

YOU
GOT
THIS

My most memorable moment of the week was . . .

_____

_____

_____

_____

_____

_____

_____

month: ....

DAY/	CYCLE DAY/

CYCLE PHASE:

☐ Menstrual

☐ Follicular

☐ Ovulatory

☐ Luteal

MOON PHASE:

Cervical Mucus:
check 'yes' or 'no' in boxes below

⬭ yes   ⬭ no

	yes	no
Tacky		
Crumbly		
Rubbery		
Creamy		
White		
Slippery		
Stringy		
Stretchy (highly fertile)		
Dry		

Bleeding/Spotting

none ☐   light ☐   medium ☐   heavy ☐

symptoms
....

☐ Cramps/Aches & Pains

☐ Headaches/Brain fog

☐ Lack of concentration

☐ Breast tenderness

☐ Nausea

☐ Loss of appetite

☐ Fatigue

☐ Insomnia

☐ Other:

ovulation?
☐ Yes   ☐ No

OVARIAN PAIN/CYSTS(which side?):

_____

BASAL BODY TEMPERATURE:

_____

☐ Regular ☐ Bloated ☐ Constipated ☐ Gassy

overall mood:

(happy) (energetic) (well–rested) (calm) (sad)

(irritable) (depressed) (anxious) (wired) (tired)

STRESS LEVEL/	*low*	*medium*	*high*
SEX or LIBIDO/	*low*	*medium*	*high*

SLEEP QUALITY	**SUPPLEMENTS:**

Nourishing Foods: _____

_____

Cravings: _____

_____

Exercise/Movement: _____

_____

_____

Workflow/Motivation: _____

_____

_____

month: ....

DAY/	CYCLE DAY/

CYCLE PHASE:

- ☐ Menstrual
- ☐ Follicular
- ☐ Ovulatory
- ☐ Luteal

MOON PHASE:

Cervical Mucus:
check 'yes' or 'no' in boxes below

	yes	no
Tacky		
Crumbly		
Rubbery		
Creamy		
White		
Slippery		
Stringy		
Stretchy (highly fertile)		
Dry		

Bleeding/Spotting

none ☐ light ☐ medium ☐ heavy ☐

symptoms
....

- ☐ Cramps/Aches & Pains
- ☐ Headaches/Brain fog
- ☐ Lack of concentration
- ☐ Breast tenderness
- ☐ Nausea
- ☐ Loss of appetite
- ☐ Fatigue
- ☐ Insomnia
- ☐ Other:

ovulation?
☐ Yes   ☐ No

OVARIAN PAIN/CYSTS(which side?):
_____

BASAL BODY TEMPERATURE:
_____

☐ Regular ☐ Bloated ☐ Constipated ☐ Gassy

overall mood:

| happy | energetic | well-rested | calm | sad |
| irritable | depressed | anxious | wired | tired |

STRESS LEVEL/	low	medium	high
SEX or LIBIDO/	low	medium	high

SLEEP QUALITY	**SUPPLEMENTS:**

Nourishing Foods: _____

_____

Cravings: _____

_____

Exercise/Movement: _____

_____

_____

Workflow/Motivation: _____

_____

_____

month: ....

DAY/	CYCLE DAY/

CYCLE PHASE:

- ☐ Menstrual
- ☐ Follicular
- ☐ Ovulatory
- ☐ Luteal

MOON PHASE:

Cervical Mucus:
check 'yes' or 'no' in boxes below

⬭ yes ⬭ no

	yes	no
Tacky		
Crumbly		
Rubbery		
Creamy		
White		
Slippery		
Stringy		
Stretchy (highly fertile)		
Dry		

Bleeding/Spotting

none ☐ light ☐ medium ☐ heavy ☐

symptoms
....

- ☐ Cramps/Aches & Pains
- ☐ Headaches/Brain fog
- ☐ Lack of concentration
- ☐ Breast tenderness
- ☐ Nausea
- ☐ Loss of appetite
- ☐ Fatigue
- ☐ Insomnia
- ☐ Other:

ovulation?

☐ Yes   ☐ No

OVARIAN PAIN/CYSTS(which side?):

_____

BASAL BODY TEMPERATURE:

_____

☐ Regular   ☐ Bloated   ☐ Constipated   ☐ Gassy

overall mood:

| happy | energetic | well-rested | calm | sad |

| irritable | depressed | anxious | wired | tired |

| **STRESS LEVEL/** | low | medium | high |
| **SEX or LIBIDO/** | low | medium | high |

SLEEP QUALITY

SUPPLEMENTS:

Nourishing Foods: _____

_____

Cravings: _____

_____

Exercise/Movement: _____

_____

_____

Workflow/Motivation: _____

_____

_____

month: ....

DAY/	CYCLE DAY/

CYCLE PHASE:

- ☐ Menstrual
- ☐ Follicular
- ☐ Ovulatory
- ☐ Luteal

MOON PHASE:

Cervical Mucus:
check 'yes' or 'no' in boxes below   (yes)   (no)

	yes	no
Tacky		
Crumbly		
Rubbery		
Creamy		
White		
Slippery		
Stringy		
Stretchy (highly fertile)		
Dry		

Bleeding/Spotting

none ☐ light ☐ medium ☐ heavy ☐

symptoms

- ☐ Cramps/Aches & Pains
- ☐ Headaches/Brain fog
- ☐ Lack of concentration
- ☐ Breast tenderness
- ☐ Nausea
- ☐ Loss of appetite
- ☐ Fatigue
- ☐ Insomnia
- ☐ Other:

ovulation?
☐ Yes   ☐ No

OVARIAN PAIN/CYSTS(which side?):

_____

BASAL BODY TEMPERATURE:

_____

Digestion:

☐ Regular   ☐ Bloated   ☐ Constipated   ☐ Gassy

overall mood:

(happy)   (energetic)   (well-rested)   (calm)   (sad)

(irritable)   (depressed)   (anxious)   (wired)   (tired)

STRESS LEVEL/	low	medium	high
SEX or LIBIDO/	low	medium	high

SLEEP QUALITY	SUPPLEMENTS:

Nourishing Foods: _____

_____

Cravings: _____

_____

Exercise/Movement: _____

_____

_____

Workflow/Motivation: _____

_____

_____

month: ....

DAY/	CYCLE DAY/

CYCLE PHASE:

- ☐ Menstrual
- ☐ Follicular
- ☐ Ovulatory
- ☐ Luteal

MOON PHASE:

Cervical Mucus:
check 'yes' or 'no' in boxes below

(yes) (no)

	yes	no
Tacky		
Crumbly		
Rubbery		
Creamy		
White		
Slippery		
Stringy		
Stretchy (highly fertile)		
Dry		

Bleeding/Spotting

none ☐   light ☐   medium ☐   heavy ☐

symptoms
....

- ☐ Cramps/Aches & Pains
- ☐ Headaches/Brain fog
- ☐ Lack of concentration
- ☐ Breast tenderness
- ☐ Nausea
- ☐ Loss of appetite
- ☐ Fatigue
- ☐ Insomnia
- ☐ Other:

ovulation?
☐ Yes   ☐ No

OVARIAN PAIN/CYSTS(which side?):
_____

BASAL BODY TEMPERATURE:
_____

Digestion:

☐ Regular ☐ Bloated ☐ Constipated ☐ Gassy

overall mood:

(happy) (energetic) (well-rested) (calm) (sad)

(irritable) (depressed) (anxious) (wired) (tired)

STRESS LEVEL/	low	medium	high
SEX or LIBIDO/	low	medium	high

SLEEP QUALITY	SUPPLEMENTS:

Nourishing Foods: _____

_____

Cravings: _____

_____

Exercise/Movement: _____

_____

_____

Workflow/Motivation: _____

_____

_____

month: ....

DAY/	CYCLE DAY/

CYCLE PHASE:

- ☐ Menstrual
- ☐ Follicular
- ☐ Ovulatory
- ☐ Luteal

MOON PHASE:

Cervical Mucus:
check 'yes' or 'no' in boxes below   (yes) (no)

	yes	no
Tacky		
Crumbly		
Rubbery		
Creamy		
White		
Slippery		
Stringy		
Stretchy (highly fertile)		
Dry		

Bleeding/Spotting

none ☐   light ☐   medium ☐   heavy ☐

symptoms
....

- ☐ Cramps/Aches & Pains
- ☐ Headaches/Brain fog
- ☐ Lack of concentration
- ☐ Breast tenderness
- ☐ Nausea
- ☐ Loss of appetite
- ☐ Fatigue
- ☐ Insomnia
- ☐ Other:

ovulation?
☐ Yes   ☐ No

OVARIAN PAIN/CYSTS(which side?):
_____

BASAL BODY TEMPERATURE:
_____

Digestion:

☐ Regular ☐ Bloated ☐ Constipated ☐ Gassy

overall mood:

happy	energetic	well-rested	calm	sad
irritable	depressed	anxious	wired	tired

STRESS LEVEL/	*low*	*medium*	*high*
SEX or LIBIDO/	*low*	*medium*	*high*

SLEEP QUALITY	**SUPPLEMENTS:**

Nourishing Foods: _____

Cravings: _____

Exercise/Movement: _____

Workflow/Motivation: _____

month: ....

DAY/	CYCLE DAY/

CYCLE PHASE:

- ☐ Menstrual
- ☐ Follicular
- ☐ Ovulatory
- ☐ Luteal

MOON PHASE:

Cervical Mucus:
check 'yes' or 'no' in boxes below   (yes) (no)

	yes	no
Tacky		
Crumbly		
Rubbery		
Creamy		
White		
Slippery		
Stringy		
Stretchy (highly fertile)		
Dry		

Bleeding/Spotting

none ☐ light ☐ medium ☐ heavy ☐

symptoms
....

- ☐ Cramps/Aches & Pains
- ☐ Headaches/Brain fog
- ☐ Lack of concentration
- ☐ Breast tenderness
- ☐ Nausea
- ☐ Loss of appetite
- ☐ Fatigue
- ☐ Insomnia
- ☐ Other:

ovulation?
☐ Yes   ☐ No

OVARIAN PAIN/CYSTS(which side?):

_____

BASAL BODY TEMPERATURE:

_____

☐ Regular   ☐ Bloated   ☐ Constipated   ☐ Gassy

overall mood:

| happy | energetic | well-rested | calm | sad |

| irritable | depressed | anxious | wired | tired |

| **STRESS LEVEL/** | low | medium | high |
| **SEX or LIBIDO/** | low | medium | high |

| **SLEEP QUALITY** | **SUPPLEMENTS:** |
| | |

Nourishing Foods: _____

_____

Cravings: _____

_____

Exercise/Movement: _____

_____

_____

Workflow/Motivation: _____

_____

_____

weekly reflection:

....

SKIN FLUCTUATIONS:

☐ Normal

☐ Oily

☐ Dry

☐ Blemishes

☐ Dull

☐ Glowy

Trying to drink more water? Meal plan? Limit social media?

. . .

Record your weekly habits here.

↓

Happy Weekly Habits: _____

_____

_____

_____

_____

_____

_____

What worked well this week?	*What did not work well this week?*

me time moments.

Record any special self-care practices like meditation, gratitude journaling, epsom salt bath, manicure... whatever "me time" means to you.

Me Time Moments: _____

_____
_____
_____
_____
_____
_____
_____
_____

YOU GOT THIS

My most memorable moment of the week was . . .

_____
_____
_____
_____
_____
_____
_____
_____

month: ....

DAY/	CYCLE DAY/

CYCLE PHASE:	MOON PHASE:
☐ Menstrual ☐ Follicular ☐ Ovulatory ☐ Luteal	

Cervical Mucus: ⬭ yes ⬭ no
check 'yes' or 'no' in boxes below

Tacky		
Crumbly		
Rubbery		
Creamy		
White		
Slippery		
Stringy		
Stretchy (highly fertile)		
Dry		

Bleeding/Spotting

none ☐ light ☐ medium ☐ heavy ☐

symptoms
....

☐ Cramps/Aches & Pains

☐ Headaches/Brain fog

☐ Lack of concentration

☐ Breast tenderness

☐ Nausea

☐ Loss of appetite

☐ Fatigue

☐ Insomnia

☐ Other:

ovulation?
☐ Yes   ☐ No

OVARIAN PAIN/CYSTS(which side?):
_____

BASAL BODY TEMPERATURE:
_____

☐ Regular ☐ Bloated ☐ Constipated ☐ Gassy

overall mood:

happy	energetic	well-rested	calm	sad
irritable	depressed	anxious	wired	tired

STRESS LEVEL/	*low*	*medium*	*high*
SEX or LIBIDO/	*low*	*medium*	*high*

SLEEP QUALITY	**SUPPLEMENTS:**

Nourishing Foods: _____

Cravings: _____

Exercise/Movement: _____

Workflow/Motivation: _____

month: ....

DAY/	CYCLE DAY/

CYCLE PHASE:

- ☐ Menstrual
- ☐ Follicular
- ☐ Ovulatory
- ☐ Luteal

MOON PHASE:

Cervical Mucus: ⬭ yes ⬭ no
check 'yes' or 'no' in boxes below

	yes	no
Tacky		
Crumbly		
Rubbery		
Creamy		
White		
Slippery		
Stringy		
Stretchy (highly fertile)		
Dry		

Bleeding/Spotting

none ☐   light ☐   medium ☐   heavy ☐

symptoms
....

- ☐ Cramps/Aches & Pains
- ☐ Headaches/Brain fog
- ☐ Lack of concentration
- ☐ Breast tenderness
- ☐ Nausea
- ☐ Loss of appetite
- ☐ Fatigue
- ☐ Insomnia
- ☐ Other:

ovulation?
☐ Yes   ☐ No

OVARIAN PAIN/CYSTS(which side?):

_____

BASAL BODY TEMPERATURE:

_____

Digestion:

☐ Regular ☐ Bloated ☐ Constipated ☐ Gassy

overall mood:

(happy) (energetic) (well-rested) (calm) (sad)

(irritable) (depressed) (anxious) (wired) (tired)

STRESS LEVEL/	low	medium	high
SEX or LIBIDO/	low	medium	high

SLEEP QUALITY	SUPPLEMENTS:

Nourishing Foods: _____

Cravings: _____

Exercise/Movement: _____

Workflow/Motivation: _____

month: ....

DAY/	CYCLE DAY/

CYCLE PHASE:

- ☐ Menstrual
- ☐ Follicular
- ☐ Ovulatory
- ☐ Luteal

MOON PHASE:

Cervical Mucus:
check 'yes' or 'no' in boxes below

	yes	no
Tacky		
Crumbly		
Rubbery		
Creamy		
White		
Slippery		
Stringy		
Stretchy (highly fertile)		
Dry		

Bleeding/Spotting

none ☐   light ☐   medium ☐   heavy ☐

symptoms
....

- ☐ Cramps/Aches & Pains
- ☐ Headaches/Brain fog
- ☐ Lack of concentration
- ☐ Breast tenderness
- ☐ Nausea
- ☐ Loss of appetite
- ☐ Fatigue
- ☐ Insomnia
- ☐ Other:

ovulation?

☐ Yes   ☐ No

OVARIAN PAIN/CYSTS(which side?):
_____

BASAL BODY TEMPERATURE:
_____

☐ Regular   ☐ Bloated   ☐ Constipated   ☐ Gassy

overall mood:

happy	energetic	well-rested	calm	sad

irritable	depressed	anxious	wired	tired

STRESS LEVEL/	low	medium	high
SEX or LIBIDO/	low	medium	high

SLEEP QUALITY	**SUPPLEMENTS:**

Nourishing Foods: _____

Cravings: _____

Exercise/Movement: _____

Workflow/Motivation: _____

month:

DAY/	CYCLE DAY/

CYCLE PHASE:

- ☐ Menstrual
- ☐ Follicular
- ☐ Ovulatory
- ☐ Luteal

MOON PHASE:

Cervical Mucus:
check 'yes' or 'no' in boxes below

	yes	no
Tacky		
Crumbly		
Rubbery		
Creamy		
White		
Slippery		
Stringy		
Stretchy (highly fertile)		
Dry		

Bleeding/Spotting

none ☐ light ☐ medium ☐ heavy ☐

symptoms

- ☐ Cramps/Aches & Pains
- ☐ Headaches/Brain fog
- ☐ Lack of concentration
- ☐ Breast tenderness
- ☐ Nausea
- ☐ Loss of appetite
- ☐ Fatigue
- ☐ Insomnia
- ☐ Other:

ovulation?

☐ Yes   ☐ No

OVARIAN PAIN/CYSTS(which side?):

BASAL BODY TEMPERATURE:

☐ Regular ☐ Bloated ☐ Constipated ☐ Gassy

overall mood:

(happy) (energetic) (well-rested) (calm) (sad)

(irritable) (depressed) (anxious) (wired) (tired)

STRESS LEVEL/	low	medium	high
SEX or LIBIDO/	low	medium	high

SLEEP QUALITY	**SUPPLEMENTS:**

Nourishing Foods: _____

_____

Cravings: _____

_____

Exercise/Movement: _____

_____

_____

Workflow/Motivation: _____

_____

_____

month: ....

DAY/	CYCLE DAY/

CYCLE PHASE:

- ☐ Menstrual
- ☐ Follicular
- ☐ Ovulatory
- ☐ Luteal

MOON PHASE:

Cervical Mucus:

check 'yes' or 'no' in boxes below   (yes) (no)

	yes	no
Tacky		
Crumbly		
Rubbery		
Creamy		
White		
Slippery		
Stringy		
Stretchy (highly fertile)		
Dry		

Bleeding/Spotting

none ☐   light ☐   medium ☐   heavy ☐

symptoms
....

- ☐ Cramps/Aches & Pains
- ☐ Headaches/Brain fog
- ☐ Lack of concentration
- ☐ Breast tenderness
- ☐ Nausea
- ☐ Loss of appetite
- ☐ Fatigue
- ☐ Insomnia
- ☐ Other:

ovulation?

☐ Yes   ☐ No

OVARIAN PAIN/CYSTS(which side?):

BASAL BODY TEMPERATURE:

☐ Regular   ☐ Bloated   ☐ Constipated   ☐ Gassy

overall mood:

(happy)   (energetic)   (well-rested)   (calm)   (sad)

(irritable)   (depressed)   (anxious)   (wired)   (tired)

STRESS LEVEL/	low	medium	high
SEX or LIBIDO/	low	medium	high

SLEEP QUALITY	**SUPPLEMENTS:**

Nourishing Foods: _____

Cravings: _____

Exercise/Movement: _____

Workflow/Motivation: _____

month: ....

DAY/	CYCLE DAY/

CYCLE PHASE:

- ☐ Menstrual
- ☐ Follicular
- ☐ Ovulatory
- ☐ Luteal

MOON PHASE:

Cervical Mucus:
☐ yes ☐ no

check 'yes' or 'no' in boxes below

Tacky		
Crumbly		
Rubbery		
Creamy		
White		
Slippery		
Stringy		
Stretchy (highly fertile)		
Dry		

Bleeding/Spotting

none ☐ light ☐ medium ☐ heavy ☐

symptoms

....

- ☐ Cramps/Aches & Pains
- ☐ Headaches/Brain fog
- ☐ Lack of concentration
- ☐ Breast tenderness
- ☐ Nausea
- ☐ Loss of appetite
- ☐ Fatigue
- ☐ Insomnia
- ☐ Other:

ovulation?

☐ Yes   ☐ No

OVARIAN PAIN/CYSTS(which side?):

_____

BASAL BODY TEMPERATURE:

_____

☐ Regular ☐ Bloated ☐ Constipated ☐ Gassy

overall mood:

| happy | energetic | well-rested | calm | sad |
| irritable | depressed | anxious | wired | tired |

| **STRESS LEVEL/** | *low* | *medium* | *high* |
| **SEX or LIBIDO/** | *low* | *medium* | *high* |

SLEEP QUALITY

SUPPLEMENTS:

Nourishing Foods: _____

Cravings: _____

Exercise/Movement: _____

Workflow/Motivation: _____

month: ....

DAY/	CYCLE DAY/

CYCLE PHASE:

- ☐ Menstrual
- ☐ Follicular
- ☐ Ovulatory
- ☐ Luteal

MOON PHASE:

Cervical Mucus:
check 'yes' or 'no' in boxes below ⬭ yes ⬭ no

	yes	no
Tacky		
Crumbly		
Rubbery		
Creamy		
White		
Slippery		
Stringy		
Stretchy (highly fertile)		
Dry		

Bleeding/Spotting

none ☐ light ☐ medium ☐ heavy ☐

symptoms
....

- ☐ Cramps/Aches & Pains
- ☐ Headaches/Brain fog
- ☐ Lack of concentration
- ☐ Breast tenderness
- ☐ Nausea
- ☐ Loss of appetite
- ☐ Fatigue
- ☐ Insomnia
- ☐ Other:

ovulation?
☐ Yes ☐ No

OVARIAN PAIN/CYSTS(which side?):
_____

BASAL BODY TEMPERATURE:
_____

Digestion:

☐ Regular ☐ Bloated ☐ Constipated ☐ Gassy

overall mood:

| happy | energetic | well-rested | calm | sad |

| irritable | depressed | anxious | wired | tired |

STRESS LEVEL/	low	medium	high
SEX or LIBIDO/	low	medium	high

SLEEP QUALITY

SUPPLEMENTS:

Nourishing Foods: _____

Cravings: _____

Exercise/Movement: _____

Workflow/Motivation: _____

weekly reflection:

SKIN FLUCTUATIONS:

- ☐ Normal
- ☐ Oily
- ☐ Dry
- ☐ Blemishes
- ☐ Dull
- ☐ Glowy

Trying to drink more water? Meal plan? Limit social media?

. . .

Record your weekly habits here.

↓

Happy Weekly Habits: _____

_____

_____

_____

_____

_____

_____

What worked well this week?	*What did not work well this week?*

me time moments.

Record any special self-care practices like meditation,
gratitude journaling, epsom salt bath, manicure...
whatever "me time" means to you.

Me Time Moments: _____

_____

_____

_____

_____

_____

_____

_____

YOU
GOT
THIS

My most memorable moment of the week was . . .

_____

_____

_____

_____

_____

_____

_____

month: ....

DAY/	CYCLE DAY/

CYCLE PHASE:

- ☐ Menstrual
- ☐ Follicular
- ☐ Ovulatory
- ☐ Luteal

MOON PHASE:

Cervical Mucus:
check 'yes' or 'no' in boxes below

	yes	no
Tacky		
Crumbly		
Rubbery		
Creamy		
White		
Slippery		
Stringy		
Stretchy (highly fertile)		
Dry		

Bleeding/Spotting

none ☐ light ☐ medium ☐ heavy ☐

symptoms

- ☐ Cramps/Aches & Pains
- ☐ Headaches/Brain fog
- ☐ Lack of concentration
- ☐ Breast tenderness
- ☐ Nausea
- ☐ Loss of appetite
- ☐ Fatigue
- ☐ Insomnia
- ☐ Other:

ovulation?
☐ Yes   ☐ No

OVARIAN PAIN/CYSTS(which side?):
_____

BASAL BODY TEMPERATURE:
_____

☐ Regular ☐ Bloated ☐ Constipated ☐ Gassy

overall mood:

(happy) (energetic) (well-rested) (calm) (sad)

(irritable) (depressed) (anxious) (wired) (tired)

STRESS LEVEL/	low	medium	high
SEX or LIBIDO/	low	medium	high

SLEEP QUALITY	SUPPLEMENTS:

Nourishing Foods: _____

Cravings: _____

Exercise/Movement: _____

Workflow/Motivation: _____

month: ....

DAY/	CYCLE DAY/

CYCLE PHASE:	MOON PHASE:
☐ Menstrual	
☐ Follicular	
☐ Ovulatory	
☐ Luteal	

Cervical Mucus:
check 'yes' or 'no' in boxes below

	yes	no
Tacky		
Crumbly		
Rubbery		
Creamy		
White		
Slippery		
Stringy		
Stretchy (highly fertile)		
Dry		

Bleeding/Spotting

none ☐ light ☐ medium ☐ heavy ☐

symptoms
....

☐ Cramps/Aches & Pains

☐ Headaches/Brain fog

☐ Lack of concentration

☐ Breast tenderness

☐ Nausea

☐ Loss of appetite

☐ Fatigue

☐ Insomnia

☐ Other:

ovulation?
☐ Yes   ☐ No

OVARIAN PAIN/CYSTS(which side?):
_____

BASAL BODY TEMPERATURE:
_____

Digestion:

☐ Regular ☐ Bloated ☐ Constipated ☐ Gassy

overall mood:

(happy) (energetic) (well-rested) (calm) (sad)

(irritable) (depressed) (anxious) (wired) (tired)

STRESS LEVEL/	low	medium	high
SEX or LIBIDO/	low	medium	high

SLEEP QUALITY	SUPPLEMENTS:

Nourishing Foods: _____

_____

Cravings: _____

_____

Exercise/Movement: _____

_____

Workflow/Motivation: _____

_____

_____

month: ....

DAY/	CYCLE DAY/

CYCLE PHASE:

- ☐ Menstrual
- ☐ Follicular
- ☐ Ovulatory
- ☐ Luteal

MOON PHASE:

Cervical Mucus:
⬭ yes ⬭ no
check 'yes' or 'no' in boxes below

	yes	no
Tacky		
Crumbly		
Rubbery		
Creamy		
White		
Slippery		
Stringy		
Stretchy (highly fertile)		
Dry		

Bleeding/Spotting

none ☐   light ☐   medium ☐   heavy ☐

symptoms
....

- ☐ Cramps/Aches & Pains
- ☐ Headaches/Brain fog
- ☐ Lack of concentration
- ☐ Breast tenderness
- ☐ Nausea
- ☐ Loss of appetite
- ☐ Fatigue
- ☐ Insomnia
- ☐ Other:

ovulation?
☐ Yes   ☐ No

OVARIAN PAIN/CYSTS(which side?):

BASAL BODY TEMPERATURE:

☐ Regular   ☐ Bloated   ☐ Constipated   ☐ Gassy

overall mood:

(happy)   (energetic)   (well-rested)   (calm)   (sad)

(irritable)   (depressed)   (anxious)   (wired)   (tired)

STRESS LEVEL/	low	medium	high
SEX or LIBIDO/	low	medium	high

SLEEP QUALITY	**SUPPLEMENTS:**

Nourishing Foods: _____

_____

Cravings: _____

_____

Exercise/Movement: _____

_____

_____

Workflow/Motivation: _____

_____

_____

month: ....

DAY/	CYCLE DAY/

CYCLE PHASE:

- ☐ Menstrual
- ☐ Follicular
- ☐ Ovulatory
- ☐ Luteal

MOON PHASE:

Cervical Mucus: ⬭ yes ⬭ no
check 'yes' or 'no' in boxes below

	yes	no
Tacky		
Crumbly		
Rubbery		
Creamy		
White		
Slippery		
Stringy		
Stretchy (highly fertile)		
Dry		

Bleeding/Spotting

none ☐ light ☐ medium ☐ heavy ☐

symptoms
....

- ☐ Cramps/Aches & Pains
- ☐ Headaches/Brain fog
- ☐ Lack of concentration
- ☐ Breast tenderness
- ☐ Nausea
- ☐ Loss of appetite
- ☐ Fatigue
- ☐ Insomnia
- ☐ Other:

ovulation?
☐ Yes ☐ No

OVARIAN PAIN/CYSTS(which side?):

_____

BASAL BODY TEMPERATURE:

_____

☐ Regular ☐ Bloated ☐ Constipated ☐ Gassy

overall mood:

happy	energetic	well-rested	calm	sad
irritable	depressed	anxious	wired	tired

STRESS LEVEL/	low	medium	high
SEX or LIBIDO/	low	medium	high

SLEEP QUALITY

SUPPLEMENTS:

Nourishing Foods: _____

_____

Cravings: _____

_____

Exercise/Movement: _____

_____

_____

Workflow/Motivation: _____

_____

_____

month: ....

DAY/	CYCLE DAY/

CYCLE PHASE:

- ☐ Menstrual
- ☐ Follicular
- ☐ Ovulatory
- ☐ Luteal

MOON PHASE:

Cervical Mucus:
check 'yes' or 'no' in boxes below

	yes	no
Tacky		
Crumbly		
Rubbery		
Creamy		
White		
Slippery		
Stringy		
Stretchy (highly fertile)		
Dry		

Bleeding/Spotting

none ☐   light ☐   medium ☐   heavy ☐

symptoms
....

- ☐ Cramps/Aches & Pains
- ☐ Headaches/Brain fog
- ☐ Lack of concentration
- ☐ Breast tenderness
- ☐ Nausea
- ☐ Loss of appetite
- ☐ Fatigue
- ☐ Insomnia
- ☐ Other:

ovulation?
☐ Yes   ☐ No

OVARIAN PAIN/CYSTS(which side?):
_____

BASAL BODY TEMPERATURE:
_____

Digestion:

☐ Regular ☐ Bloated ☐ Constipated ☐ Gassy

overall mood:

(happy) (energetic) (well-rested) (calm) (sad)

(irritable) (depressed) (anxious) (wired) (tired)

STRESS LEVEL/	low	medium	high
SEX or LIBIDO/	low	medium	high

SLEEP QUALITY	SUPPLEMENTS:

Nourishing Foods: _____

Cravings: _____

Exercise/Movement: _____

Workflow/Motivation: _____

month: ....

DAY/	CYCLE DAY/

CYCLE PHASE:

- ❏ Menstrual
- ❏ Follicular
- ❏ Ovulatory
- ❏ Luteal

MOON PHASE:

Cervical Mucus: ⬭ yes ⬭ no
check 'yes' or 'no' in boxes below

	yes	no
Tacky		
Crumbly		
Rubbery		
Creamy		
White		
Slippery		
Stringy		
Stretchy (highly fertile)		
Dry		

Bleeding/Spotting

none ❏ light ❏ medium ❏ heavy ❏

symptoms

- ❏ Cramps/Aches & Pains
- ❏ Headaches/Brain fog
- ❏ Lack of concentration
- ❏ Breast tenderness
- ❏ Nausea
- ❏ Loss of appetite
- ❏ Fatigue
- ❏ Insomnia
- ❏ Other:

ovulation?
❏ Yes   ❏ No

OVARIAN PAIN/CYSTS(which side?):
_____

BASAL BODY TEMPERATURE:
_____

☐ Regular ☐ Bloated ☐ Constipated ☐ Gassy

overall mood:

(happy) (energetic) (well-rested) (calm) (sad)

(irritable) (depressed) (anxious) (wired) (tired)

STRESS LEVEL/	low	medium	high
SEX or LIBIDO/	low	medium	high

SLEEP QUALITY	SUPPLEMENTS:

Nourishing Foods: _____

Cravings: _____

Exercise/Movement: _____

Workflow/Motivation: _____

month: ....

DAY/	CYCLE DAY/

CYCLE PHASE:	**MOON PHASE:**

CYCLE PHASE:

- ☐ Menstrual
- ☐ Follicular
- ☐ Ovulatory
- ☐ Luteal

MOON PHASE:

Cervical Mucus: ⬭ yes ⬭ no
check 'yes' or 'no' in boxes below

	yes	no
Tacky		
Crumbly		
Rubbery		
Creamy		
White		
Slippery		
Stringy		
Stretchy (highly fertile)		
Dry		

Bleeding/Spotting

none ☐ light ☐ medium ☐ heavy ☐

symptoms
....

- ☐ Cramps/Aches & Pains
- ☐ Headaches/Brain fog
- ☐ Lack of concentration
- ☐ Breast tenderness
- ☐ Nausea
- ☐ Loss of appetite
- ☐ Fatigue
- ☐ Insomnia
- ☐ Other:

ovulation?
☐ Yes ☐ No

OVARIAN PAIN/CYSTS(which side?):
_____

BASAL BODY TEMPERATURE:
_____

Digestion:

☐ Regular ☐ Bloated ☐ Constipated ☐ Gassy

overall mood:

(happy) (energetic) (well-rested) (calm) (sad)

(irritable) (depressed) (anxious) (wired) (tired)

STRESS LEVEL/	low	medium	high
SEX or LIBIDO/	low	medium	high

SLEEP QUALITY	SUPPLEMENTS:

Nourishing Foods: _____

_____

Cravings: _____

_____

Exercise/Movement: _____

_____

_____

Workflow/Motivation: _____

_____

_____

weekly reflection:

SKIN FLUCTUATIONS:

☐ Normal

☐ Oily

☐ Dry

☐ Blemishes

☐ Dull

☐ Glowy

Trying to drink more water? Meal plan? Limit social media?

. . .

Record your weekly habits here.

↓

Happy Weekly Habits: _____

_____

_____

_____

_____

_____

_____

What worked well this week?	*What did not work well this week?*

me time moments.

Record any special self-care practices like meditation, gratitude journaling, epsom salt bath, manicure... whatever "me time" means to you.

Me Time Moments: _____

_____

_____

_____

_____

_____

_____

_____

_____

YOU
GOT
THIS

My most memorable moment of the week was . . .

_____

_____

_____

_____

_____

_____

_____

_____

month: ....

DAY/	CYCLE DAY/

CYCLE PHASE:

☐ Menstrual

☐ Follicular

☐ Ovulatory

☐ Luteal

MOON PHASE:

Cervical Mucus: ⬭ yes   ⬭ no
check 'yes' or 'no' in boxes below

	yes	no
Tacky		
Crumbly		
Rubbery		
Creamy		
White		
Slippery		
Stringy		
Stretchy (highly fertile)		
Dry		

Bleeding/Spotting

none ☐   light ☐   medium ☐   heavy ☐

symptoms
....

☐   Cramps/Aches & Pains

☐   Headaches/Brain fog

☐   Lack of concentration

☐   Breast tenderness

☐   Nausea

☐   Loss of appetite

☐   Fatigue

☐   Insomnia

☐   Other:

ovulation?
☐ Yes   ☐ No

OVARIAN PAIN/CYSTS(which side?):

_____

BASAL BODY TEMPERATURE:

_____

☐ Regular ☐ Bloated ☐ Constipated ☐ Gassy

overall mood:

| happy | energetic | well-rested | calm | sad |
| irritable | depressed | anxious | wired | tired |

| **STRESS LEVEL/** | *low* | *medium* | *high* |
| **SEX or LIBIDO/** | *low* | *medium* | *high* |

SLEEP QUALITY	**SUPPLEMENTS:**

Nourishing Foods: _____

Cravings: _____

Exercise/Movement: _____

Workflow/Motivation: _____

month: ....

DAY/	CYCLE DAY/

CYCLE PHASE:

- ☐ Menstrual
- ☐ Follicular
- ☐ Ovulatory
- ☐ Luteal

MOON PHASE:

Cervical Mucus:
check 'yes' or 'no' in boxes below   ⬭ yes   ⬭ no

	yes	no
Tacky		
Crumbly		
Rubbery		
Creamy		
White		
Slippery		
Stringy		
Stretchy (highly fertile)		
Dry		

Bleeding/Spotting

none ☐ light ☐ medium ☐ heavy ☐

symptoms
....

- ☐ Cramps/Aches & Pains
- ☐ Headaches/Brain fog
- ☐ Lack of concentration
- ☐ Breast tenderness
- ☐ Nausea
- ☐ Loss of appetite
- ☐ Fatigue
- ☐ Insomnia
- ☐ Other:

ovulation?
☐ Yes   ☐ No

OVARIAN PAIN/CYSTS(which side?):
_____

BASAL BODY TEMPERATURE:
_____

Digestion:

☐ Regular ☐ Bloated ☐ Constipated ☐ Gassy

overall mood:

(happy) (energetic) (well-rested) (calm) (sad)

(irritable) (depressed) (anxious) (wired) (tired)

STRESS LEVEL/	low	medium	high
SEX or LIBIDO/	low	medium	high

SLEEP QUALITY

SUPPLEMENTS:

Nourishing Foods: _____

Cravings: _____

Exercise/Movement: _____

Workflow/Motivation: _____

month: ....

DAY/	CYCLE DAY/

CYCLE PHASE:

- ☐ Menstrual
- ☐ Follicular
- ☐ Ovulatory
- ☐ Luteal

MOON PHASE:

Cervical Mucus:
check 'yes' or 'no' in boxes below   (yes)   (no)

	yes	no
Tacky		
Crumbly		
Rubbery		
Creamy		
White		
Slippery		
Stringy		
Stretchy (highly fertile)		
Dry		

Bleeding/Spotting

none ☐   light ☐   medium ☐   heavy ☐

symptoms
....

- ☐ Cramps/Aches & Pains
- ☐ Headaches/Brain fog
- ☐ Lack of concentration
- ☐ Breast tenderness
- ☐ Nausea
- ☐ Loss of appetite
- ☐ Fatigue
- ☐ Insomnia
- ☐ Other:

ovulation?
☐ Yes   ☐ No

OVARIAN PAIN/CYSTS(which side?):
_____

BASAL BODY TEMPERATURE:

Digestion:

☐ Regular ☐ Bloated ☐ Constipated ☐ Gassy

overall mood:

(happy) (energetic) (well-rested) (calm) (sad)

(irritable) (depressed) (anxious) (wired) (tired)

STRESS LEVEL/	low	medium	high
SEX or LIBIDO/	low	medium	high

SLEEP QUALITY	SUPPLEMENTS:

Nourishing Foods: _____

_____

Cravings: _____

_____

Exercise/Movement: _____

_____

_____

Workflow/Motivation: _____

_____

_____

month: ....

DAY/	CYCLE DAY/

CYCLE PHASE:

☐ Menstrual
☐ Follicular
☐ Ovulatory
☐ Luteal

MOON PHASE:

Cervical Mucus:
check 'yes' or 'no' in boxes below

(yes) (no)

	yes	no
Tacky		
Crumbly		
Rubbery		
Creamy		
White		
Slippery		
Stringy		
Stretchy (highly fertile)		
Dry		

Bleeding/Spotting

none ☐ light ☐ medium ☐ heavy ☐

symptoms
....

☐ Cramps/Aches & Pains
☐ Headaches/Brain fog
☐ Lack of concentration
☐ Breast tenderness
☐ Nausea
☐ Loss of appetite
☐ Fatigue
☐ Insomnia
☐ Other:

ovulation?
☐ Yes   ☐ No

OVARIAN PAIN/CYSTS(which side?):
_____

BASAL BODY TEMPERATURE:
_____

Digestion:

☐ Regular ☐ Bloated ☐ Constipated ☐ Gassy

overall mood:

happy	energetic	well-rested	calm	sad
irritable	depressed	anxious	wired	tired

STRESS LEVEL/	low	medium	high
SEX or LIBIDO/	low	medium	high

SLEEP QUALITY	**SUPPLEMENTS:**

Nourishing Foods: _____

Cravings: _____

Exercise/Movement: _____

Workflow/Motivation: _____

month: ....

DAY/	CYCLE DAY/

CYCLE PHASE:	*MOON PHASE:*

CYCLE PHASE:

- ☐ Menstrual
- ☐ Follicular
- ☐ Ovulatory
- ☐ Luteal

MOON PHASE:

Cervical Mucus: ⟨yes⟩ ⟨no⟩
check 'yes' or 'no' in boxes below

	yes	no
Tacky		
Crumbly		
Rubbery		
Creamy		
White		
Slippery		
Stringy		
Stretchy (highly fertile)		
Dry		

Bleeding/Spotting

none ☐　light ☐　medium ☐　heavy ☐

symptoms
....

- ☐ Cramps/Aches & Pains
- ☐ Headaches/Brain fog
- ☐ Lack of concentration
- ☐ Breast tenderness
- ☐ Nausea
- ☐ Loss of appetite
- ☐ Fatigue
- ☐ Insomnia
- ☐ Other:

ovulation?
☐ Yes　　☐ No

OVARIAN PAIN/CYSTS(which side?):
_____

BASAL BODY TEMPERATURE:
_____

☐ Regular ☐ Bloated ☐ Constipated ☐ Gassy

overall mood:

happy	energetic	well-rested	calm	sad
irritable	depressed	anxious	wired	tired

STRESS LEVEL/	low	medium	high
SEX or LIBIDO/	low	medium	high

SLEEP QUALITY	SUPPLEMENTS:

Nourishing Foods: _____

_____

Cravings: _____

_____

Exercise/Movement: _____

_____

_____

Workflow/Motivation: _____

_____

_____

month: ....

DAY/	CYCLE DAY/

CYCLE PHASE:

- ☐ Menstrual
- ☐ Follicular
- ☐ Ovulatory
- ☐ Luteal

MOON PHASE:

Cervical Mucus: ⬭yes ⬭no
check 'yes' or 'no' in boxes below

Tacky		
Crumbly		
Rubbery		
Creamy		
White		
Slippery		
Stringy		
Stretchy (highly fertile)		
Dry		

Bleeding/Spotting

none ☐   light ☐   medium ☐   heavy ☐

symptoms

- ☐ Cramps/Aches & Pains
- ☐ Headaches/Brain fog
- ☐ Lack of concentration
- ☐ Breast tenderness
- ☐ Nausea
- ☐ Loss of appetite
- ☐ Fatigue
- ☐ Insomnia
- ☐ Other:

ovulation?

☐ Yes   ☐ No

OVARIAN PAIN/CYSTS(which side?):
_____

BASAL BODY TEMPERATURE:
_____

Digestion:

☐ Regular ☐ Bloated ☐ Constipated ☐ Gassy

overall mood:

happy	energetic	well-rested	calm	sad
irritable	depressed	anxious	wired	tired

STRESS LEVEL/	low	medium	high
SEX or LIBIDO/	low	medium	high

SLEEP QUALITY	**SUPPLEMENTS:**

Nourishing Foods: _____

Cravings: _____

Exercise/Movement: _____

Workflow/Motivation: _____

month: ....

DAY/	CYCLE DAY/

CYCLE PHASE:

- ☐ Menstrual
- ☐ Follicular
- ☐ Ovulatory
- ☐ Luteal

MOON PHASE:

Cervical Mucus:
check 'yes' or 'no' in boxes below

(yes) (no)

	yes	no
Tacky		
Crumbly		
Rubbery		
Creamy		
White		
Slippery		
Stringy		
Stretchy (highly fertile)		
Dry		

Bleeding/Spotting

none ☐   light ☐   medium ☐   heavy ☐

symptoms
....

- ☐ Cramps/Aches & Pains
- ☐ Headaches/Brain fog
- ☐ Lack of concentration
- ☐ Breast tenderness
- ☐ Nausea
- ☐ Loss of appetite
- ☐ Fatigue
- ☐ Insomnia
- ☐ Other:

ovulation?

☐ Yes   ☐ No

OVARIAN PAIN/CYSTS(which side?):
_____

BASAL BODY TEMPERATURE:
_____

☐ Regular ☐ Bloated ☐ Constipated ☐ Gassy

overall mood:

| happy | energetic | well-rested | calm | sad |

| irritable | depressed | anxious | wired | tired |

STRESS LEVEL/	*low*	*medium*	*high*
SEX or LIBIDO/	*low*	*medium*	*high*

SLEEP QUALITY	**SUPPLEMENTS:**

Nourishing Foods: _____

_____

Cravings: _____

_____

Exercise/Movement: _____

_____

_____

Workflow/Motivation: _____

_____

_____

weekly reflection:

SKIN FLUCTUATIONS:

☐ Normal

☐ Oily

☐ Dry

☐ Blemishes

☐ Dull

☐ Glowy

Trying to drink more water? Meal plan? Limit social media?

. . .

Record your weekly habits here.

↓

Happy Weekly Habits: _____

_____

_____

_____

_____

_____

_____

What worked well this week?

What did not work well this week?

me time moments.

Record any special self-care practices like meditation,
gratitude journaling, epsom salt bath, manicure...
whatever "me time" means to you.

Me Time Moments: _____
_____
_____
_____
_____
_____
_____
_____
_____
_____

YOU
GOT
THIS

My most memorable moment
of the week was . . .

_____
_____
_____
_____
_____
_____
_____
_____
_____

about the author:

Shannon Leparski is the founder, photographer, wellness blogger, and recipe developer behind The Glowing Fridge, a vibrant blog where she promotes living a plant-based vegan lifestyle. Her lifelong passion for wellness, green beauty, and nutrition began in high school and through her undergraduate years at Purdue University. The Glowing Fridge has transformed into a plant-fueled resource, allowing Shannon to do what she loves: create vibrant recipes and holistic-based content focused around optimal health and hormone balance. She has inspired thousands to transition toward a plant-forward life! Shannon's first book, *The Happy Hormone Guide*, presents a comprehensive, plant-based lifestyle program to help women balance their hormones, increase energy, and reduce PMS symptoms. Shannon resides in the northwest suburbs of Chicago with her chihuahua (Taz) and husband (Terry).

Published by Blue Star Press
PO Box 8835, Bend, OR 97708
contact@bluestarpress.com
www.bluestarpress.com

Design by Megan Kesting

ISBN: 9781950968176

Printed in China

10 9 8 7 6 5 4 3 2 1

DISCLAIMER:
This book is for informational and educational purposes only. Please
consult your healthcare provider before beginning any healthcare program.